Doppler Ultrasound in Gynecology

PROGRESS IN OBSTETRIC
AND GYNECOLOGICAL
SONOGRAPHY SERIES

SERIES EDITOR: ASIM KURJAK

Doppler Ultrasound in Gynecology

Edited by

A. KURJAK and A. C. FLEISCHER

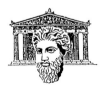

The Parthenon Publishing Group
International Publishers in Medicine, Science & Technology

NEW YORK   LONDON

Library of Congress Cataloging-in-Publication Data

Doppler ultrasound in gynecology/edited by
  A. Kurjak and A. C. Fleischer.
     p. cm.—(Progress in obstetric and
gynecological sonography series)
   Includes bibliographical references and index.
   ISBN 1-85070-623-9
   1. Doppler ultrasonography. 2.
Generative organs, Female—Ultrasonic imaging.
   I. Kurjak, Asim. II. Fleischer, Arthur C.
   III. Series.
     [DNLM: 1. Genital Diseases. Female—
ultrasonography. 2. Ultrasonography.
Doppler—methods.   WP 141 D691 1997]
RG107.5.U4D67 1997
618.1′07543—dc21
DNLM/DLC
for Library of Congress   97-41399
                                                      CIP

British Library Cataloguing in Publication Data

Doppler ultrasound in gynecology.—(Progress in
  obstetric and gynecological sonography series)
     1. Doppler ultrasonography 2. Generative
  organs, Female—Ultrasonic imaging
     3. Ultrasonics in obstetrics
  I. Kurjak, Asim   II. Fleischer, Arthur C.
  618′.04′7543
     ISBN 1-85070-623-9

Published in the USA by
The Parthenon Publishing Group Inc.
One Blue Hill Plaza
PO Box 1564, Pearl River
New York 10965, USA

Published in the UK and Europe by
The Parthenon Publishing Group Limited
Casterton Hall, Carnforth
Lancs. LA6 2LA, UK

Copyright © 1998 Parthenon Publishing Group

First published 1998

Typeset by AMA Graphics Ltd., Preston,
Lancashire, UK
Printed and bound in Spain by
T. G. Hostench, S. A.

Contents

List of principal contributors

A. C. Fleischer
Department of Radiology and Radiological
  Sciences
Vanderbilt University Medical Center
CCC-1121 Medical Center North
1161 21st Avenue, South Nashville
TN 37232-2675
USA

S. Fujiwaki
Department of Obstetrics and Gynecology
St. Marianna University, School of Medicine
2-16-1 Sugao
Miyamae-ku, Kawasaki City
216 Japan

S. Kupesic
Department of Obstetrics and Gynecology
Medical School University of Zagreb
Sveti Duh Hospital
Sveti Duh 64
10000 Zagreb
Croatia

A. Kurjak
Department of Obstetrics and Gynecology
Medical School University of Zagreb
Sveti Duh Hospital
Sveti Duh 64
10000 Zagreb
Croatia

L. Valentin
Department of Obstetrics and Gynecology
Malmo University Hospital
S-205 02 Malmo
Sweden

H. Yun
Jersey City Medical Center
Department of Obstetrics and Gynecology
Jersey City, New Jersey
USA

I. Žalud
Department of Obstetrics and Gynecology
Winthrop University Hospital
259 First Street
Mineola, New York 11501
USA

Foreword

Color Doppler sonography has become extensively utilized for the evaluation of certain gynecological disorders. It affords physiological as well as anatomic assessment. Color Doppler sonography continues to expand into new applications, realizing that it also has limitations.

The technique is no longer in its infancy. Controversies exist and are welcome in order to promote a critical and objective evaluation. There are many objective and subjective reasons for this situation, for example, the low reliability of results and their reproducibility, the high technical complexity, inadequate education and knowledge about pelvic hemodynamics, a lack of standardization in Doppler measurements, cost–benefit issues (Doppler machines are usually very expensive), the question of whether Doppler should be used as a screening tool or as a secondary or even tertiary test, the interpretation of results, the time taken for the procedure, and the question of safety in early pregnancy. Certainly, more time is needed to answer the current questions and dilemmas.

This monograph contains up-to-date information regarding the clinical use of Doppler sonography as well as admission of its limitations. It is hoped that this information may be helpful to those who use and refer patients for this diagnostic modality.

Asim Kurjak
Arther C. Fleischer

Accuracy, precision and artifacts of Doppler measurements in gynecology

1

I. Žalud, B. Breyer and A. Kurjak

The Doppler technique has been used in medicine for many years, but only in the last decade has this diagnostic modality gained importance in obstetrics, and then gradually in gynecology. Conventional and very well-established B-mode ultrasound gives information about morphology. Doppler ultrasound gives information about blood flow, and at the same time some 'functional' aspects of the observed anatomical structure. Ultrasound is now able not only to answer the question 'What is this structure on the ultrasound screen?', but also to answer some questions about how this structure is behaving. Ultrasound is a unique diagnostic modality, combining anatomical and functional information.

The potential for Doppler ultrasound applications in gynecology is tremendous but unfortunately still not very well explored. Information obtained by Doppler could help in better diagnosis and treatment of many old gynecological problems. However, despite tremendous effort and research interest from all around the world, particularly from Europe, the USA, Japan and Israel, promising results from Doppler research are still far from practical and routine clinical application. There are many objective and subjective reasons for this situation, such as: low result reliability and reproducibility, high technical complexity, inadequate education and knowledge of pelvic hemodynamics, lack of standardization in Doppler measurements, cost–benefit issues (Doppler machines are usually very expensive), the question of whether Doppler should be used as a screening tool or as a secondary or even tertiary test, interpretation of results, time taken for the procedure, question of safety in early pregnancy, etc.

Doppler in gynecology has been particularly of interest since transvaginal color Doppler sonography was introduced in 1986. The major issues in this field are screening for pelvic malignancy (ovarian carcinoma in the first instance), more accurate preoperative diagnosis of pelvic masses and selection of an adequate surgical approach, diagnostic help in gynecological emergencies such as ectopic pregnancy or ovarian torsion, help in the diagnosis and treatment of infertility, selection of candidates for an *in vitro* fertilization embryo transfer (IVF–ET) program, etc. Although there are more than 100 publications every year quoted in Medline, Doppler as a diagnostic tool in gynecology is still very far from routine clinical application. One of the major reasons for so many conflicting and controversial results in the literature originates from the complexity of the technique and inadequate education.

For intelligent and successful application of the technique to medical diagnosis, an understanding of Doppler physics, its possibilities and limitations is necessary. Flow can be detected even in vessels that are too small to image. Doppler ultrasound can determine the presence or absence of flow, flow direction and flow character. One of the fundamental limitations of flow information provided by Doppler is that it is angle dependent. Furthermore, artifacts in Doppler ultrasound can be confusing and lead to misinterpretation of flow information. These problems will be addressed in this chapter.

The basic principle of the Doppler effect for the case when the waves reflect from a reflector is illustrated in Figure 1. If the reflector does not move (case a) the frequency of the reflected wave f_1 is equal to the transmitted frequency f_0.

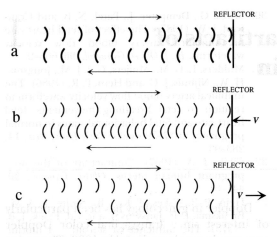

Figure 1 Basic principle of the Doppler effect

Ultrasound waves   Scatterers

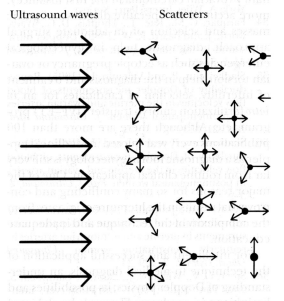

Figure 2 Ultrasound scatters on blood cells

If the reflector moves towards the transceiver (case b), the reflected frequency will be higher than the transmitted frequency. If the reflector moves away (case c) from the transceiver, the received frequency f_1 will be lower than the transmitted frequency f_0. This frequency change Δf (called the Doppler shift) is proportional to the velocity v of the reflector movement.

In practice, this means that we need an apparatus that transmits ultrasound waves into the body and receives their reflections from the

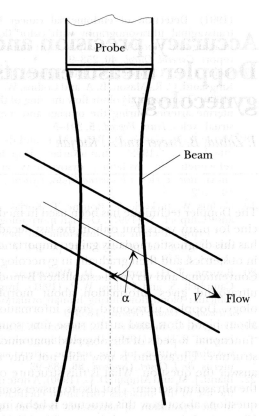

Figure 3 Illustration of the angle (α) between the ultrasound beam and the flow

body. The apparatus must then measure the difference between the transmitted and received frequencies. The frequency difference (Doppler shift expressed in Hertz) is proportional to the velocity of the movement along the line that connects the wave transceiver and the moving reflector.

In medical applications, the Doppler effect is usually measured by insonating the moving blood and assessing the Doppler shift of ultrasound scattered by erythrocytes (Figure 2). Single erythrocytes reflect (retransmit) ultrasound in various directions, but the back-scattered energy is sufficient for velocity assessment.

The general method of measurement consists of transmission of bundled ultrasound into the body at a general angle α to the flow (Figure 3). In this case, the following equation of Doppler shift is valid to a sufficient approximation:

$$\Delta f = \frac{2f_0 V}{c} \cos \alpha$$

It is important to note that in this approximation the Doppler shift for $\alpha = 90°$ equals zero.

A more detailed theory shows that for wave beams the Doppler shift is not exactly zero at $\alpha = 90°$, but the shift is small and not used in the present commercial instrumentation. Thus the plane wave approximation from the above equation is valid for normal practice[1,2].

From the above Doppler shift formula, we can calculate the velocity (m/s) by the equation:

$$V = \frac{\Delta f \times c}{2f_0 \cos \alpha}$$

with c = ultrasound propagation speed, Δf = Doppler shift, f_0 = transmitted wave frequency, and α the angle between the ultrasound beam and the flow direction.

The flow in blood vessels depends on the quality of their walls and vessel dimensions. If the flow is laminar (when the walls are even and the blood vessel is large enough), the flow profile is parabolic, that is, the velocity in the center is the fastest and slows down as we approach the walls (Figure 4). If there is an obstacle in the blood vessel (a plaque, a branching, etc.) the profile deviates from a parabola and can become turbulent. In any case, at any instance at any cross-section, the blood flows at many different velocities at the same time, i.e. there is a full spectrum of flow velocities. The results are usually shown as Doppler shift spectra in real time, as in Figure 5.

The ordinate is the Doppler shift (Figures 5 and 6) and the abscissa is the running time. Doppler shift measured in Hertz is proportional to flow velocity and, if the angle α is known, one can put velocities onto the ordinate by using the above equation. The upper spectrum (ART) has the typical shape of an arterial spectrum. It is

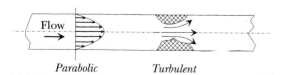

Figure 4 Normal and disturbed flow

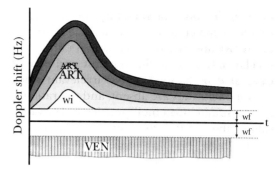

Figure 5 Arterial spectrum (ART) is pulsatile, while the peripheral vein spectrum (VEN) is fairly continuous. wf, wall filter

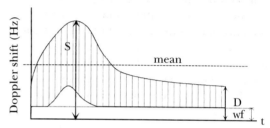

Figure 6 Resistance and pulsatility indices are calculated using the peak velocities at peak systole (S) and at end-diastole (D). wf, wall filter

pulsatile. The venous spectrum (VEN) in the lower part of Figure 5 is not pulsatile. Since the blood flows at each instance at different velocities, the spectra are generally filled in. The lowest frequencies are cut off with special high-pass filters, the so-called wall filters (wf). The filter was originally designed to eliminate the artifacts from moving blood vessel walls.

Apart from absolute velocity measurement, one can define relative indices, which are particularly useful for flow evaluation without a known angle between the flow and the ultrasound beam.

DOPPLER INDICES

Because of inherent difficulties in evaluating blood flow, or even in accepting depicted velocities as accurate, the blood flow velocity waveform has commonly been interpreted to distinguish patterns associated with high and low resistance in the distal vascular tree (Figure 6). Three indices are in common use: the systolic/diastolic ratio (S/D ratio), the pulsatility index (PI, also called the impedance index) and the resistance index (RI, also called the Pourcelot ratio).

The S/D ratio is the simplest and can be calculated by hand, but it is irrelevant when diastolic velocities are absent, and the ratio becomes infinite. Common practice has grouped values above 8.0 into a single category 'extremely high'.

The PI requires computer-assisted calculation of mean velocity, which still may be subject to very large experimental error. In a normal pregnancy, neither the S/D ratio nor the PI is normally distributed across all gestational ages.

The RI is moderately complicated, but has the appeal of approaching 1.00 when diastolic velocities are abnormally low and does, therefore, reflect the relative impairment of flow by high resistance. These indices are ratios, independent of the angle between the ultrasound beam and the insonated blood vessel, and therefore not dependent on absolute measurement of true velocity.

The indices were derived initially by their statistically demonstrated association with adverse clinical findings. They are commonly regarded as 'resistance indices', reflecting the belief that they indicate the degree of downstream resistance. However, the RI must not be considered to be independent of changes in physiological variables such as heart rate, cardiac contractility, blood pressure and the many other determinants of flow. This information does not depend on the measurement angle, since all the parts of the spectrum change proportionally when the angle α changes. However, as the angle approaches 90°, the measurement error increases rapidly. In practice, the best compromise between the resolution of the B-mode image and the accuracy of Doppler spectroscopy is obtained at angles between 30 and 60°.

The three indices are highly correlated, with coefficients in excess of 0.9 being reported[3,4]. Such is the degree of correlation that it is unlikely that one index provides an advantage over the other. There are intrinsic errors in all that have been quantified and lie between 10 and 20%. There may be advantages to the RI or PI where flow is markedly abnormal or in early pregnancy, when a very low end-diastolic velocity can be a normal finding. Given the many modifications and adaptations proposed in the literature, use of a particular index becomes a matter of personal choice. Formulae for the indices are as follows:

$$\text{Resistance index,} \quad RI = \frac{S - D}{S}$$

$$\text{Pulsatility index,} \quad PI = \frac{S - D}{\text{mean}}$$

INSTRUMENTATION FOR DOPPLER MEASUREMENTS

There are two basic technological methods for application of the Doppler effect in medicine (Figure 7). It is possible to transmit and receive ultrasound waves continuously with a probe that contains a transmission transducer and a reception transducer (CW in Figure 7). Another possibility is to transmit in the form of pulses whose Doppler shift is measured after the time necessary for ultrasound to reach a defined depth in the body (PW in Figure 7). These two systems have different properties (Table 1).

The CW system has no depth resolution, so that the measurements of all flows along the line of sight add together and mix. On the other hand, this system makes good measurements of all (fast and slow) velocities. If there is only one blood vessel along the line of sight or one flow is dominant, the CW system is useful for practice.

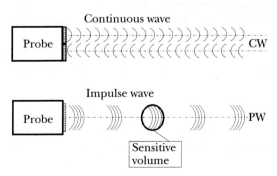

Figure 7 Illustration of continuous wave and pulsed wave Doppler measurement methods

Table 1 Comparison of different types of Doppler instruments

Type	Advantage	Disadvantage	Other
Spectrometers			
Pulsed wave	has depth resolution	poorly measures high velocities deep in the body	higher price
High pulse rate frequency system	PW system which can measure fast flows	ambiguous measurement (multiple sensitive volumes)	requires more caution from operator
Continuous wave	measures all velocities	has no depth resolution – mixes flows along the us. beam	lower price
Two-dimensional Doppler systems			
'Color Doppler'	yields the directional flow map and indication of turbulence	does not measure at 90°, less sensitive than spectrometer	quite sensitive to incorrect manipulation
'Power Doppler'	sensitive to small flows, does not confuse the operator with unclear direction data	poorly follows fast flow changes	unknown clinical usefulness

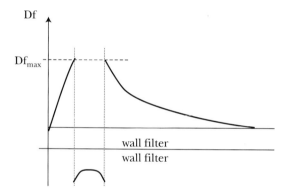

Figure 8 Aliasing causes the velocities that are too high to be shown as opposite flow. Df, Doppler shift

If, however, one must measure the flow in a single blood vessel, the pulsed wave system can measure within a sensitive volume. The sensitive volume has a length that depends on the pulse length (in time) and a width that depends on the beam width (and focusing) (shown later in Figure 9). The disadvantage of such a pulse Doppler system is that it cannot measure high velocities deep in the body. The reason for this is that a pulsed wave system only occasionally looks at the flow, so that it cannot convey all the information at a high enough throughput. The phenomenon can mathematically be described by the sampling theorem, which results in aliasing, i.e. reverse indication of flow that is too fast.

(The resulting artifact is shown in Figures 8, 11 and 13.)

The top of the pulsatile spectrum (highest velocities) is shown as negative (reverse flow). If the spectrum is simple, as in Figure 8, the recognition of the aliasing artifact is easy. In complex spectra this can be difficult. In such cases it may be useful to have a combined pulsed wave and continuous wave system or a high pulse rate frequency system. This system has such a pulse rate that it violates the sampling theorem and thus yields mathematically ambiguous results. On the screen, this is usually shown as multiple sampling volumes (spots, cursors). Such a system measures at multiple spots at a time. If the operator can recognize the spots with dominant flow or position the cursors in such a way that only one of them hits flow, the system achieves a better performance for high-velocity flow measurement.

DATA ACQUISITION

The computerized generation of the flow velocity waveform is not a simple task (Table 2). In addition to the loss of returned frequencies by random scattering and tissue attenuation, a number of computer-based steps are required to eliminate low-frequency noise generated by tissues vibrating in response to the ultrasound

Table 2 Ultrasound modalities

Modality	Medium/dimension
Two-dimensional ultrasound	echo location
	echo amplitude
Pulsed Doppler	Doppler shift
Color Doppler	echo location
	Doppler shift
Power Doppler	echo amplitude
	echo location
Time-domain ultrasound	echo location
	time shift

beam and by non-ultrasound-based movement of tissues, and high-frequency emissions of the transducer itself, not to mention the complexities of the echoes that are returned as a result of blood flow.

Several mechanisms are used to 'clean up' the returned frequencies. Their inherent liabilities will be noted.

Low-pass filtering (only frequencies below a set limit are displayed) eliminates high-frequency instrument noise. Although some information is lost, this usually does not interfere with biological Doppler application.

High-pass filtering (to be used in the display, frequencies must be above a set minimum that is usually able to be regulated by the operator) removes unwanted low-frequency signals. Thus, interference from vessel wall vibration, or other tissue movement, is eliminated – but this mechanism will also remove low velocities representing low flow. High-pass filtering, therefore, is capable of erroneously suggesting absent flow in diastole.

The sample volume (or 'range gate') limits the area to be analyzed. In duplex scanning, the range gate is adjustable for width and for position. Range-gating assumes a standard time interval between pulse emission and echo return, based on the standard tissue transmit time from the depth set by the operator. The receiving gate is open only for the anticipated moment of echo return, thus restricting information received to what is 'expected' from the area designated by the calipers on the screen. While limiting Doppler data to the area requested, this mechanism has an important stipulation: the sample volume should be larger than the vessel, and positioned

to span it completely. If it is set too large, extraneous signals may be included.

These mechanisms, therefore, restrict the information that is returned and analyzed, in an effort to refine the waveform and present an acceptable image. Clearly, this 'editing' has the potential to omit desirable (usually low) velocities.

SIGNAL PROCESSING

Since only a small fraction of the transmitted ultrasound is reflected in the direction of the transducer, substantial amplification is required. The data are then purified by the combination of filtration and demodulation. Demodulation consists of comparing the standard generated carrier frequencies of the transducer's output, to determine shifted frequencies, Doppler shifted echoes within the spatial domain of the ultrasound beam and conforming to the known ranges typical of physiological flow speeds from the raw data generated by the purification process. The final step in this process is separation according to direction of flow, with output from the phase quadrature detector in two channels, flow toward the transducer represented as a positive Doppler shift and flow away from the transducer represented as a negative Doppler shift. The next step in the presentation of a flow image is the organization of the purified data into a depiction of Doppler shift changes over time.

The process of Doppler spectral analysis involves sorting the various velocities and displaying them in a ranked format. The digital analytical method used to order the Doppler spectrum from low to high velocities on the vertical axis is the fast Fourier transform. This process uses sine wave modelling to sort out the various velocity components of the received signal in real time. Ultimately, this is displayed on the screen as a blood flow velocity waveform.

FLOW VS. VELOCITY

The display is of velocity vs. time. The theoretical steps in the calculation of velocity have already been noted, but there are several problems in

Table 3 Factors influencing blood flow

Pressure

Myocardial function
Preload, afterload
Valvular competence
Vessel tone (vasomotor status)
Tissue characteristics

Resistance

Cross-sectional outflow area
Blood viscosity
Metabolic state
Vessel length
Vessel geometry (branching, stenosis)
Vessel characteristics (elastic impedance)

accepting the blood flow velocity 'in centimeters per second' as a literal value. First, measurement of the Doppler angle is actually quite difficult. In fetal echocardiography, the beam is assumed to be parallel to the direction of flow and the Doppler angle does not matter (Doppler angle = 0°, cos 0° = 1.00). A final group of concerns is the natural inclination to make statements about flow based on the depiction of velocities. Many factors may affect blood flow (Table 3). Further, the nature of the flow (pulsatile or steady, regular or turbulent, single or branching, parabolic or plug), impacts significantly on the frequencies returned. Thus, although volume blood flow can be calculated as the product of mean blood flow velocity and vessel area, this is fraught with variation in practical terms.

The cross-sectional area of the vessel measured from the gray-scale image is very susceptible to error. For a 6–8-mm vessel (e.g. iliac artery), an error of 0.4 mm in diameter produces a 10% error in calculated flow. This same measurement error for a 4-mm vessel would produce a 25% error. Pulsations in arteries, for example, produce changes in diameter that have been assessed in the iliac artery to vary as much as 20%[1,2].

Another major problem in measuring flow is the variation of blood velocity across the vessel cross-section. Because the overall flow rate is the sum of the contributions made by the blood at every point on the cross-section, it is necessary to average the velocity profile (mean blood flow velocity). Various approaches to this have been described. They can be categorized according to whether the velocity profile is measured (using multigated pulsed Doppler) and then averaged or averaged using a large sample volume to encompass the whole vessel. Volume blood flow has been expressed as milliliters per minute per kilogram. Estimating the fetal weight by ultrasound measurement formulae is also error-prone. It is clear that, to allow accurate or even moderately useful volume flow measurement, Doppler interrogation must be limited to large vessels, with meticulous attention to methodology.

Figure 8 is an illustration of the aliasing effect on an arterial spectrum where the peak velocities have been too fast to measure with the particular pulse repetition frequency (PRF) of a pulsed Doppler system.

TWO-DIMENSIONAL FLOW MEASUREMENT

Color Doppler display

The flow can be shown in two dimensions. In principle, this can be achieved by comparison or subtraction of successive two-dimensional images. Only echoes from moving structures remain in such images. The final result is a two-dimensional display of moving structures, mainly blood flowing through blood vessels.

The directions and speeds are color-coded. Movements towards the probe are shown in different shades of one color, e.g. red, and away from the probe in shades of another color, e.g. blue. The different shades signify relative velocity. One must always bear in mind that this system shows the component of velocity projected onto the probing ultrasound beam. This makes the display semiquantitative. The multiple Doppler shift measurement variance can be displayed. In the red–blue combination code, the variance is usually shown in green. The larger the measurement variance, the more green. This gives an indication of turbulence. Flow at 90° to the ultrasound beam is not shown (in the image it is shown as black, i.e. as if it were

7

Table 4 Differences between normal color Doppler and power Doppler

Color Doppler	Power Doppler
Shows direction	insensitive to direction
Brightness proportional to velocity	brightness shows quantity of moving blood
Color angle-dependent	color angle-independent
Color independent of depth	color depth-dependent (and adjustable)
Moderate sensitivity	high sensitivity
Has aliasing artifacts	no aliasing
Sensitive to probe movement	sensitive to probe movement
Interpretation requires much knowledge	simpler interpretation with fewer data
Critical sensitivity manipulation	not very critical sensitivity manipulation
Can yield elaborate velocity information	little velocity information
Two-dimensional display gives a clue about the type of flow (faster image renewal)	gives little clue about the type of flow (very slow image repetition)
Large clinical experience already exists	little clinical experience

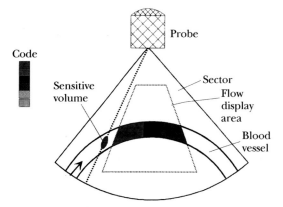

Figure 9 Two-dimensional mapping of flow uses color maps to represent flow direction and color brightness to represent the velocity

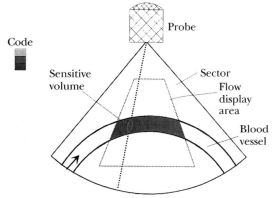

Figure 10 'Power Doppler' is a representation method in which only the existence of flow is shown in different hues of one color

not there). The color code is arbitrary and in the majority of machines can be chosen from a number of different possibilities. Since the two-dimensional color Doppler is semiquantitative, it is usually combined with a pulsed wave Doppler spectrometer. The two-dimensional display helps in fast finding of the points where we wish to analyze the flow by spectrometry. In this way the two-dimensional system reduces the duration of Doppler examinations. Sometimes, however, the two-dimensional map is characteristic enough to help with the diagnosis. The limitations of the method are the same as those of the pulse Doppler technique, and so we now have the ubiquitous 'color Doppler' (Figure 9). As with any new method, the first amazement has yielded to systematic and often controversial,

but always tedious, evaluation in clinical medicine. Since many of the most feared illnesses develop on a long time scale, the method is still under scrutiny, but is already accepted as a useful tool. A particular form of two-dimensional flow mapping is called power Doppler (Figure 10).

Power Doppler ultrasound

The shortcomings of the two-dimensional directional Doppler ('color Doppler') are many (Table 4). Above all, the sensitivity to direction is a mixed blessing. It does give the much valued information about the direction of flow, but suffers from not very high sensitivity and direction artifacts. In many cases the directional information is very valuable, as in echocardiography. However, there are many instances when the only relevant question is 'Where are the blood vessels?' or 'How many blood vessels are there?' or 'What is the perfusion of this area?'. The direction may be of little importance or determinable with a built-in Doppler spectrometer. Color Doppler yields that information. However, it is not uncommon to find a clear Doppler spectrum signal from an area that is completely without any color signal or where (if we are lucky) the color appears occasionally. The reason for this is that the directional information is evaluated from a number of subsequent frames and ambiguous and low signals average out to zero.

All these considerations led the instrumentation researchers to take a step backwards and develop a two-dimensional system which just detects and displays movement, any movement, in two dimensions. The result is an instrument that displays areas with moving structures in color. The color means that there is flow in the area and the brightness of the color qualitatively indicates the quantity of moving erythrocytes.

Every normal color Doppler system has the basic capability for 'power Doppler' or 'Doppler angio'. Power Doppler is a mode of operation in which any signal that shows a Doppler shift (change in frequency) is tagged with color, so the direction becomes irrelevant. Unlike color Doppler, in which a symmetrical turbulence shows a poor signal, in power Doppler the signal will be as strong as any. The reason for this is that when directional information is displayed, the zero mean velocity is not displayed, while in the case when the total reflection from any moving structure is displayed a turbulent flow is as indicative as any.

The decision as to what is flow and what is not is taken by looking at the frequency spectra; high enough frequency shifts are considered to represent blood flow. The color coding is made proportional in brightness to the total power of reflected ultrasound from moving structures. Structures which do not move, or move slowly, are not color-coded. The displayed color indicates the quantity of moving blood, but not the volume flow of blood per unit time. The virtue of this display mode is that it shows fast and slow flow equally, so that we can get a feeling of the general blood perfusion in an area. However, if actual blood velocity or volume per unit time is of interest, we must revert to other display and measurement modes.

The flow display in this case depends on the total 'power', a signal proportional to the average reflected amplitude. This depends on the density of red blood cells within the ultrasound sampling volume. The returned signal depends, in addition, on the attenuation of ultrasound in the intervening tissue. This means that the flow in deeper blood vessels or the flow in the same blood vessel that changes depth will be shown with different brightness, depending on the depth.

The density of the moving blood cells depends on the concentration of blood cells and the local flow situation. The sampling volume depends on the length of the ultrasound pulse and the beam width. If the sampling volume is larger than the blood vessel, the average number of red blood cells in it will be smaller and the returned signal will thus be relatively weaker, showing a dimmer color brightness on the display.

LIMITATIONS OF DOPPLER EXAMINATIONS

There exists no method without shortcomings and limitations. In Doppler measurements one encounters problems of accuracy, precision and artifacts, as in any measurement and imaging method. The peculiarities of this method are as follows.

Accuracy

Doppler spectrometry operates adequately for angles between the ultrasound beam and flow of < 60°. The theoretical measurement error tends asymptotically towards infinity when the angle approaches 90°. The raw result of the measurement is a spectrum that illustrates the general behavior well, but has the data on velocity hidden by an additional unknown factor – the angle. However, even with the angle α known, data such as mean velocity can be calculated only by way of a fairly complicated numerical integral

9

of the weighted spectrum. The mechanism that picks up the respective weights of single velocities within the spectrum at each instant operates fairly autonomously, usually without the intervention of the operator. Intervention by way of changing the measurement sensitivity can change the result of the calculation. It must continuously be borne in mind that Doppler shift only is to be measured, whereas the rest of the data are derived from this. The accuracy of assessment of the Doppler shift depends on the knowledge and control of the frequency content of the ultrasound pulses. This is often not well controlled. An exception is operation with continuous wave Doppler systems, in which the measurement can be made more accurate.

Color Doppler itself is not designed as an accurate measurement method, but mainly as a semiquantitative guiding method for Doppler shift spectroscopy. In spite of this, the significance of different colors must be known, and in particular one must carefully adjust the baseline shift, since this can essentially change the velocity–color map.

There is, however, a possibility of extracting accurate data on the Doppler shift by using a cursor, which helps in reading the frequency shift from the computer memory. Fourier power spectra, where available, give quantitative data, but these are often not well understood. This spectrum is not a real-time spectrum but a graph with the Doppler shift on the abscissa and the energy in the frequency range on the ordinate. Its width and symmetry properties contain ample information about the nature of the flow (which is harder to read from the usual real-time spectrum). This power spectrum should not be confused with 'power Doppler'.

The power Doppler display method has a slightly better geometrical accuracy in showing the blood vessel lumen than the normal 'color Doppler'. This occurs at the cost of image repetition rate.

Precision

The quantitative functional dependence of the velocity measurement error on the knowledge of the angle α is known. However, the usual method of measurement of the angle is very crude and thus one should try to avoid using absolute values whenever possible.

Since the color map scale is virtually continuous, there is only marginal accuracy in the judgement of the velocity by way of color assessment. However, the variance map, although not accurately assessable, gives a very useful clue as to where one ought to do spectroscopic measurements. Again, the Fourier power spectrum capability enables a precise variance calculation and the power Doppler modality increases observation sensitivity at the cost of losing directional information.

Artifacts

Several artifacts are encountered in Doppler ultrasound[5–10]. These arise from incorrect presentation of Doppler flow information (Table 5). The most common of these is aliasing. However, others occur, including range ambiguity, spectrum mirror image, location mirror image, speckle and electromagnetic interference.

Aliasing

Aliasing is the most common artifact encountered in Doppler ultrasound (Figures 8, 11, 12 and 13).

There is an upper limit to the Doppler shift that can be detected by pulsed instruments. If the Doppler shift frequency exceeds one-half the pulse repetition frequency (normally in the 1–30 kHz range), aliasing occurs and improper Doppler shift information (improper direction and improper value) results. An analogous optical form of aliasing occurs in motion pictures, when wagon wheels appear to rotate at various speeds and in the reverse direction. Higher pulse repetition frequencies permit higher Doppler shifts to be detected, but also increase the chance of the range ambiguity artifact. Continuous wave Doppler instruments do not have this limitation, but neither do they provide depth selectivity.

Table 5 Summary of Doppler artifacts

Error	Cause	Effect
Aliasing	high flow exceeds 0.5 pulse repetition frequency Doppler angle moving	velocity peaks switch direction: information lost biphasic flow wave
Double image	Doppler angle near 90°	wave duplicated in both directions
Mirror image	strong reflector adjacent (e.g. pelvic side wall or bone)	inappropriate gate location loss of Doppler information
Speckle	Doppler gain too high	indistinct waveform overstated peak velocity
Range ambiguity	tissue layers (e.g. large cyst) change beam velocity	aberrant depth resolution incorrect gate location
Beam deflection	tissue layers change Doppler angle	reduced lateral spatial definition incorrect gate location
Clipping	excessive wall filter gate inside vessel	loss of low velocity, misperception of high resistance

Aliasing can be eliminated by increasing the pulse repetition frequency, increasing the Doppler angle (which decreases the Doppler shift for a given flow), or by baseline shifting. The latter is an electronic 'cut and paste' technique that moves the misplaced aliasing peaks over to their proper location. It is a successful technique as long as there are no legitimate Doppler shifts in the region of the aliasing. If there are, they will get moved over to an inappropriate location along with the aliasing peaks. Other approaches to eliminating aliasing include changing to a lower-frequency Doppler transducer or changing to a continuous wave instrument. Aliasing occurs with the pulsed system because it is a sampling system. If samples are taken often enough, the correct result is achieved. Insufficient sampling yields an incorrect result.

The Nyquist limit or Nyquist frequency describes the minimum number of samples required to avoid aliasing. There must be at least two samples per cycle of the desired wave in order for it to be obtained correctly. For a complicated signal such as a Doppler signal containing many frequencies, the sampling rate must be such that at least two samples occur for each cycle of the highest frequency present. To restate this rule, if the highest Doppler shift frequency present in a signal exceeds one-half the pulse repetition frequency, aliasing will occur.

Range ambiguity

In an attempt to solve the aliasing problem by increasing pulse repetition frequency, the range ambiguity problem can be encountered. This occurs when a pulse is emitted before all the echoes from the previous pulse have been received. When this happens, early echoes from the last pulse are simultaneously received with late echoes from the previous pulse. This causes difficulty with the ranging process. The instrument is unable to determine whether an echo is an early one (superficial) from the last pulse or a late one (deep) from the previous pulse. To avoid this difficulty, it simply assumes that all echoes are derived from the last pulse and that these echoes have originated from some depth as determined by the 13 μs/cm rule. As long as all echoes are received before the next pulse is sent out, this will be true. However, with high pulse repetition frequencies, this may not be the case. Doppler flow information may, therefore, come from locations other than the assumed one (the gate location). In effect, multiple gates or sample volumes are operating at different depths. Instruments often increase pulse repetition frequency (to avoid aliasing) into the range where range ambiguity occurs. Multiple sample gates are shown on the display to indicate this condition. Range ambiguity in color flow Doppler, as in sonography, places echoes (color Doppler shifts in this case) that have come from

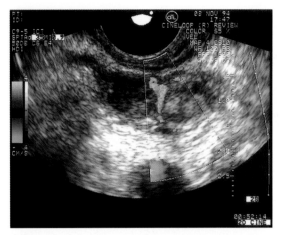

Figure 11 Color Doppler aliasing in the small pelvic vessels

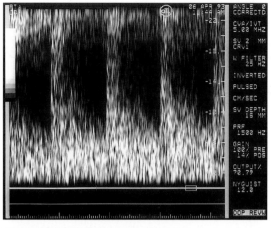

Figure 13 Pulsed Doppler aliasing

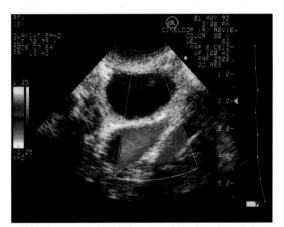

Figure 12 An example of proper color Doppler settings to avoid aliasing in the internal iliac vessels

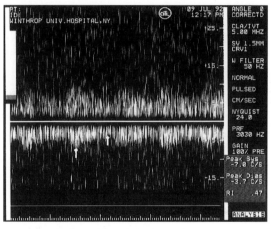

Figure 14 Mirror image artifact

deep locations after a subsequent pulse was emitted in shallow locations where they do not belong. As already stated, the high pulse rate frequency systems intentionally introduce this ambiguity for spectrometry, requiring sound judgement by the operator as to whether the results are correct or not.

Mirror images

The mirror image artifact can also occur with Doppler systems (Figure 14). This means that an image of a vessel and a source of Doppler shifted echoes can be duplicated on the opposite side of a strong reflector (such as a bone).

The duplicated vessel containing flow could be misinterpreted as an additional vessel. It will have a spectrum similar to that for the real vessel. A mirror image of a Doppler spectrum can appear on the opposite side of the baseline when, indeed, flow is unidirectional and should appear only on one side of the baseline. This is an electronic duplication of the spectral information. It can occur when receiver gain is set too high (causing overloading in the receiver and cross talk between the two flow channels) or with low gain (where the receiver has difficulty determining the sign of the Doppler shift). It can also occur when the Doppler angle is near 90°. Here the duplication is usually legitimate. This is because beams are focused and not cylindrical in shape. Thus, portions of the beam can experience flow toward while other portions can experience flow away[13].

Speckle

Doppler spectra have a speckle quality to them similar to that observed in sonography. Speckle is a result of interference effects of scattered sound from the distribution of scatterers (erythrocytes) in the blood. Because the ultrasound pulse encounters several scatterers at any point in its travel, several echoes are generated simultaneously. These may arrive at the transducer in such a way that they re-enforce (constructive interference) or partially or totally cancel (destructive interference) each other. This results in a displayed dot pattern that does not directly represent individual scatterers but rather represents an interference pattern of the scatter distribution scanned. This phenomenon is called acoustic speckle (Figure 15). It is analogous to the speckle phenomenon observed when a laser is shone on a wall.

Electromagnetic interference

Occasionally, a spectral trace can show a straight line adjacent to and parallel to the baseline, often on both sides (Figure 16). Apparently, this is due to 60-Hz interference from power lines or power supply. It can make determination of low or absent diastolic flow difficult. Electromagnetic interference from power lines and nearby equipment can also cloud the spectral display with lines or 'snow'. Improper pulse repetition frequency settings can ultimately cause erroneous diagnosis of an absent diastolic blood flow (Figures 17–19).

In Figure 5, 'wi' indicates the 'window' – an empty space in the real-time spectrum. Strictly speaking, this space ought never to be empty, but, in the case of parabolic flow and somewhat reduced sensitivity, the space will not fill with measurement results. This logic applies if the sensitive volume takes up the whole blood vessel cross-section. However, if we reduce the sensitive volume so as to take up only a small part of the blood vessel, a 'window' will appear even at fairly irregular flows. This does not much influence the assessment of RI and PI, but disturbs our assessment of the turbulence. Very turbulent flow will show at the same time a positive (towards probe) and negative (away from probe) flow spectrum. However, a similar spectrum appearance can be expected if we put the measurement angle near 90°. Therefore, we must always interpret the cause of the apparent synchronous flow in opposite directions. An additional possibility is to fit a curve of a small blood vessel in the same sample volume, which then yields opposite flows in the two parts of the 'hook' as opposite, nearly symmetrical spectra.

Inadvertent change of the wall filter can cut off the diastolic part of the arterial

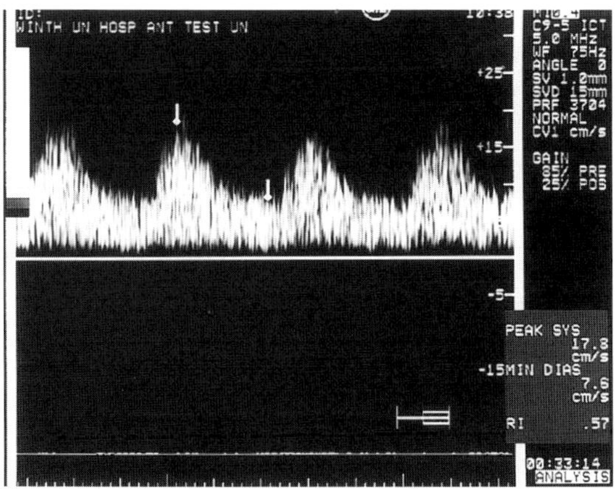

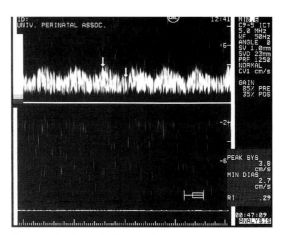

Figure 15 Acoustic speckle

Figure 16 Straight line artifact

Doppler spectrum and lead to incorrect clinical diagnosis.

How to reduce problems

(1) Use the sensitivity control (gain) with caution (use as low a sensitivity as practical);

(2) Start examination with the standard symmetrical color map and then gradually change it to non-symmetrical types if needed;

(3) Be aware of the depth and increased aliasing probability at deeper structures and higher velocities; and

(4) Use all the three modes (B-mode, spectrum and color) for survey, but use a single modality to obtain the best quality of each of them.

SAFETY

Risk and safety considerations are always of interest in medical diagnostic techniques. It is desirable to gain information that will be useful in guiding patient management, while minimizing any risk resulting from the diagnostic procedure. Biological effects of ultrasound exposure have been studied in cells, plants and experimental animals and several epidemiological studies have been performed. From this information we develop an approach to the appropriate and prudent use of Doppler ultrasound as a medical diagnostic tool.

For consideration of the safety of diagnostic ultrasound, an attempt must be made to relate knowledge of bioeffects to the clinical situation. There are three questions that arise when an attempt is made to accomplish this:

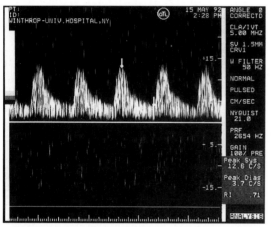

Figure 17 An example of proper setting of pulse repetition frequency (PRF) when analyzing the uterine artery blood flow velocity (PRF = 2654 Hz)

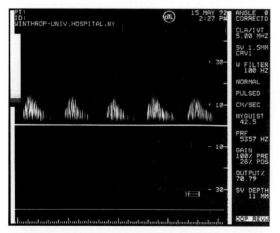

Figure 18 The same vessel as in Figure 17 analyzed at higher pulse repetition frequency (PRF). Of note is an artificial disappearance of diastolic blood flow (PRF = 5357 Hz)

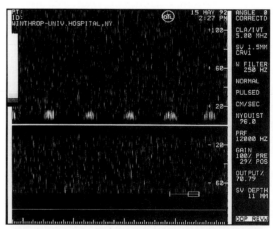

Figure 19 The same vessel as in Figures 17 and 18. High pulse repetition frequency (PRF) setting completely eliminates display of diastolic blood flow and can lead to disappearance of systolic blood flow display as well (PRF = 12000 Hz)

(1) Do any of the bioeffects that have occurred under experimental conditions constitute a hazard to a human in the clinical setting?

(2) Are the acoustic parameters at the site of the bioeffects in experimental animals comparable to those at the appropriate site of concern in the human body during diagnosis?

(3) Do the continuous wave conditions of most experimental studies provide any useful information for the pulsed ultrasound of clinical diagnosis?

These questions remain largely unanswered. As there is no satisfactory response to question 1, an attempt must be made to determine whether any bioeffects observed in experimental animals are likely to occur clinically. This brings us to the difficulties of questions 2 and 3. The response to question 2 is that in human applications of ultrasound, the organs of concern are normally farther from the sound source (a longer attenuating sound path is involved). Also, a smaller organ volume fraction is exposed because the organs are larger than those of the usual experimental animals. These considerations may provide some (unknown) safety factors for the diagnostic situation. Concerning question 3, it is not known whether or not short diagnostic pulses of low duty factor can produce bioeffects under clinical conditions and whether or not repair could occur between pulses.

In the meantime, with no known risk and known benefit to the procedure, a conservative approach to Doppler ultrasound should be used. That is, Doppler should be used when medically indicated with minimum exposure of the patient and fetus (Figure 20).

Exposure is minimized by minimizing instrument output intensity and by minimizing exposure time during a study. Experiments by one of us (B.B.) have shown that it is possible to induce water streaming with almost all commercial pulse Doppler instruments, and this confirms results obtained by others[11]. Doppler instrument outputs can be significantly higher than those for imaging. It seems most likely that the

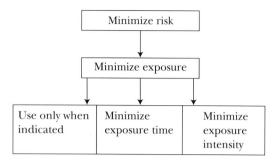

Figure 20 Safety aspects of Doppler ultrasound exposure

greatest potential for risk in ultrasound diagnosis (although no specific risk has been identified even in this case) is for fetal or embryonic studies. These combine potentially high output intensities with stationary geometry and the (presumably more sensitive) fetus. It should be emphasized that color flow imaging uses a scanning beam just as sonography does so that the potential risk situation in this case appears to be less serious than for conventional Doppler spectral analysis.

Extensive mechanistic, *in vitro*, *in vivo* and epidemiological studies have revealed no known risk with current ultrasound instrumentation used in medical diagnosis, both imaging and Doppler[12]. However, a prudent and conservative approach to ultrasound safety is to assume that there may be unidentified risks that should be minimized in medically indicated ultrasound studies by minimizing exposure time and intensity. In short, we should minimize the (unknown, but potentially non-zero) risk by minimizing exposure.

CONCLUSIONS

Doppler ultrasound is unique among clinical techniques in that Doppler has the potential to offer information related to the function of an organ beside its morphology. Before exploring the roles of Doppler ultrasound, one must consider the possibility that the information returned is erroneous. Common ways of receiving inaccurate information are listed in Table 5. Most of these errors are obvious from the display and it is likely that the custom of reporting relative indices rather than using absolute Doppler velocities reduces the significance of such errors. It seems to the authors that misinterpreting the Doppler, or making inappropriate decisions on the basis of Doppler information, is far more likely. Because of the relative novelty of gynecological Doppler under real-time ultrasound direction, standards of application have not yet evolved.

Artifacts in color and spectral Doppler imaging can be confusing and lead to misinterpretation of blood flow information. Inappropriate equipment settings, anatomical factors and physical and technical limitation of the modality are encountered as the major causes. Incorrect gain, wall-filter, or velocity scale settings can cause loss of clinically important information or distortion of the tracing. Artifacts in Doppler ultrasound include aliasing, range ambiguity, image and Doppler signal mirroring, spectral trace mirroring, and 60-Hz interference. Aliasing is the most common artifact. It occurs when the Doppler shift frequency exceeds half the pulse repetition frequency. It can be reduced or eliminated by increasing the pulse repetition frequency or Doppler angle, using baseline shift, reducing operating frequency, or using a continuous wave instrument. Recognizing these artifacts is important to avoid image misinterpretations and, when possible, to overcome them by modifying either techniques or unit settings, or both. It must be kept in mind that an accurate analysis of unit settings during scanning, and the meticulous evaluation of the obtained Doppler images are of the utmost importance for the proper use of this valuable but difficult diagnostic modality.

It is obvious that the display of color and pulsed Doppler information is a complicated and sometimes confusing technology, owing to the many controls and their interactions. Understanding what each of these controls does independently and how the image is affected by adjustment and change is essential. More importantly, a permanent awareness of which control to sacrifice and which to enhance in each specific pelvic vessel is critical in obtaining the most diagnostically useful Doppler information.

Several epidemiological studies have indicated no risk with the use of diagnostic ultrasound. Because there is limited specific knowledge, the conservative approach is taken: use diagnostic ultrasound with minimum exposure when medical benefit is expected from the procedure.

References

1. Mitchell, D. G. (1990). Color Doppler imaging: principles, limitations, and artifacts. *Radiology*, **177**, 1–10
2. Kremkau, F. W. (1992). Doppler color imaging: principles and instrumentation. *Clin. Diagn. Ultrasound*, **27**, 7–60
3. Burns, P. N. (1993). Principles of Doppler and color flow. *Radiol. Med.*, **85**, 3–16
4. Taylor, K. J. W. and Holland, S. (1990). Doppler ultrasound. Part I: Basic principles, instrumentation, and pitfalls. *Radiology*, **174**, 297–307
5. Zalud, I. and Kurjak, A. (1994). Artifacts and pitfalls. In Kurjak, A. (ed.) *Transvaginal Color Doppler*, 2nd edn, pp. 353–8. (Carnforth, UK: Parthenon Publishing)
6. Derchi, L. E., Giannoni, M., Crespi, G., Pretolesi, F. and Oliva, L. (1992). Artifacts in echo-Doppler and color-Doppler. *Radiol. Med.*, **83**, 340–52
7. Jaffe, R. (1992). Color Doppler imaging: a new interpretation of the Doppler effect. In Jaffe, R. and Warsof, S. L. (eds.) *Color Doppler Imaging in Obstetrics and Gynecology*, pp. 17–34. (New York: McGraw-Hill)
8. Winkler, P., Helmke, K. and Mahl, M. (1990). Major pitfalls in Doppler investigations. Part II: Low flow velocity and colour Doppler application. *Pediatr. Radiol.*, **20**, 304–10
9. Suchet, I. B. (1994). Colour-flow Doppler artifacts in anechoic soft-tissue masses of infants. *Can. Assoc. Radiol. J.*, **45**, 201–3

10. Pozniak, M. A., Zagzebski, J. A. and Scanlan, K. A. (1992). Spectral and color Doppler artifacts. *Radiographics,* **12**, 35–44

11. Duck, F. and Zauhar, G. (1996). Report on experiments by H. Starrit, G. Zauhar and F. Duck in Bath, autumn

12. Maulik, D. (1997). Biosafety of diagnostic Doppler ultrasonography. In Maulik, D. (ed.) *Doppler Ultrasound in Obstetrics and Gynecology,* pp. 88–106. (New York: Springer)

13. Censor, D., Newhouse, V. L. and Ortega, H. V. (1988). Theory of ultrasound Doppler spectra velocimetry for arbitrary beam and flow configurations. *IEEE Trans. Biomed. Eng.,* **35**, 740

Normal pelvic blood flow

2

S. Kupesic, A. Kurjak and M. M. Babić

Transvaginal color Doppler sonography provides a unique non-invasive method for evaluating normal and abnormal conditions in the female pelvis[1]. This method has superior accuracy and reproducibility, and enables the visualization of small vessels under physiological conditions. It is hoped that this simplified examination technique will be used as a clinical therapeutic aid, promising exciting future developments. Transvaginal color Doppler sonography affords detailed delineation of the uterus and its myometrium, endometrium and vessels[2], and gives a potential tool to the investigator to study and observe the female reproductive system and vascular changes within the pelvis. The resistance index (RI) depends on age, phase of the menstrual cycle and special conditions (such as pregnancy or utcrine tumors).

Quantification of color flow can be achieved by pulsed Doppler waveform analysis. The peak systolic (A) and end-diastolic (B) Doppler shift frequencies can be recorded, and the A/B ratio, Pourcelot resistance index, or pulsatility index (PI) may be calculated.

Therefore, blood flow in the main pelvic vessels can easily be visualized and recognized with this new modality. The transvaginal transducer clearly displays the entire vessel coursing from the sides of the cervix, up to the lateral wall of the uterus and along the Fallopian tube, to terminate above the ovaries. The artery and vein can be distinguished according to the pulsation and brightness of color flow. Iliac vessels can be seen on the side wall of the pelvis, often lying deep, close to the ovary.

Pulsed Doppler waveform analysis of an iliac artery shows high velocity and high resistance to blood flow with a characteristic normal finding of reversed flow ('triphasic pattern') (Figure 1). Both the internal and external iliac arteries have the same 'signature'. Doppler analysis shows very low-velocity blood flow in iliac veins, without the regular systolic–diastolic variation.

The iliac arteries at the bifurcation have characteristic waveforms. The common and external iliac arteries that are part of the aortofemoral segment show plug flow, a window under the waveform and a reversed component during diastole. The internal iliac artery, in contrast, has a parabolic flow with an even distribution of velocities within the waveform.

The continuous venous flow pattern can be affected by transmitted pulsation of the internal iliac artery (Figure 2). Visualization of iliac veins is an excellent way to document patency or thrombosis.

The common iliac vessels can only occasionally be seen, because they are usually too far from the probe. They present a high velocity with the most prominent reversed flow in diastole. The phenomenon of reversed flow in the iliac vessels can be explained by high peripheral resistance in the pelvis and the legs, causing blood to rebound back up to the iliac arteries and aorta.

The uterine artery originates from the internal iliac artery, whereas the ovarian artery is a direct branch of the abdominal aorta. The vascular supply to the uterus is provided by a complex network of arteries originating from the uterine artery. Its main branches extend inward for about a third of the myometrium, forming the arcuate wreath which encircles the uterus[3] (Figure 3). Smaller branches called radial arteries are directed towards the uterine lumen[4]. When they pass the inner third of the myometrium and myometrioendometrial junction, they become spiral arteries. The color Doppler signal from the main uterine artery may be seen in all patients laterally to the cervix at the level of the cervicocorporeal junction (Figure 4).

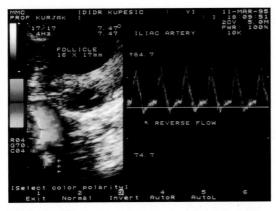

Figure 1 The internal iliac artery. The pulsed Doppler waveform analysis (right) shows high-velocity and high-resistance blood flow with the characteristic normal finding of reversed flow

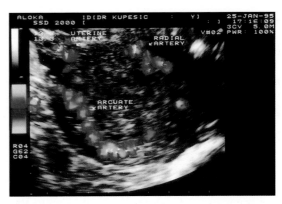

Figure 3 Uterine artery demonstrated laterally to the cervix at the level of the cervicocorporeal junction. After extending inward for about a third of the thickness of the myometrium, the uterine arteries divide into an arcuate wreath encircling the myometrium. Radial arteries arise from this network and are directed towards the uterine lumen

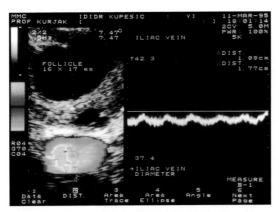

Figure 2 The internal iliac vein. The pulsed Doppler waveform analysis (right) shows very low-velocity blood flow without the regular systolic–diastolic variation. The continuous venous flow pattern is affected by transmitted pulsations of the internal iliac artery

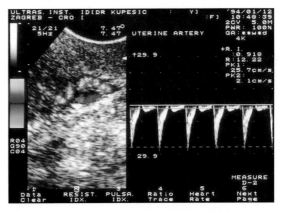

Figure 4 Blood flow velocity from the uterine artery in the proliferative phase is characterized by a small amount of end-diastolic flow and high impedance to blood flow (RI = 0.92)

Transvaginal color Doppler can be used to obtain flow velocity waveforms from the uterine arteries at any time during the menstrual cycle[5]. It is apparent that there are complex relationships between the concentration of ovarian hormones in peripheral venous plasma and uterine artery blood flow parameters[6–8] (Figure 5).

Deutinger and co-workers[9] found that ovarian steroids altered the function of periarterial sympathetic nerves through changes in α_1-adrenergic receptor numbers and led to marked changes of the blood flow. In animal studies, the injection of estradiol led to an increase of blood flow in pelvic arteries. In humans, the increase of the serum estradiol level is combined with an increase of the left ventricular end-diastolic dimension, stroke volume and cardiac index, and with a decline of the RI.

In most women, there is a small amount of end-diastolic flow in the uterine arteries during the proliferative phase. Goswamy and Steptoe[6] found increasing RI and systolic/diastolic ratio

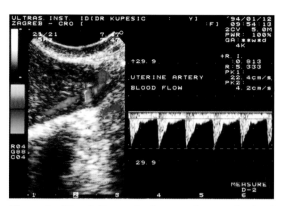

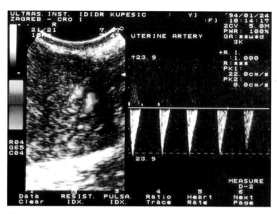

Figure 5 Blood flow velocity waveforms obtained from the uterine artery in the secretory phase characterized by increased end-diastolic velocity and decreased resistance index (RI = 0.81)

Figure 6 Pulsed Doppler signals obtained from the uterine arteries display no end-diastolic component of blood flow. This finding may be associated with infertility or poor reproductive capacity

during the postovulatory drop in the serum estradiol concentration.

During the normal menstrual cycle there is a sharp increase in end-diastolic velocities between the proliferative and secretory phases of the menstrual cycle. It is particularly interesting that the lowest blood flow impedance occurs during the time of peak luteal function, during which implantation is most likely to occur. It is logical that blood supply to the uterus should be high in the late luteal phase, as reported by Kurjak and colleagues[5], Goswamy and colleagues[6,7], Battaglia and colleagues[10] and Steer and colleagues[11]. In anovulatory cycles these changes are not present, and continuous increase in the RI is seen. In some infertile patients the end-diastolic flow is not present, indicating that poor uterine perfusion is a potential cause of infertility (Figure 6).

Scholtes and colleagues[12] used a combined transvaginal two-dimensional real-time and pulsed Doppler method for recording flow velocity waveforms in the uterine and ovarian arteries from 16 healthy women during the follicular and luteal phases of the normal menstrual cycle: on days 7, 13, 16 and 21. In contrast to earlier reports, their study displayed forward end-diastolic velocities in at least 70% of the ovarian artery flow velocity waveforms and in nearly all uterine flow velocity waveforms. If end-diastolic velocities were absent, this was

always during the early follicular stage (day 7) of the menstrual cycle. The higher percentage of absent end-diastolic blood flow velocities documented in previous studies may have been the result of methodological error, such as too large an interrogation angle between the Doppler beam and flow direction, too high a cut-off level of the high-pass filter, or too low an energy input with small sample volumes for the equipment used.

The observation that left–right differences in PI were not related to the site of ovulation suggested that there was no essential difference in blood supply to the left and right ovarian arteries. Serial assessment of the flow velocity waveforms reveals a decrease in PI from the ovarian arteries supplying the ovary carrying the dominant follicle and subsequent corpus luteum, which is statistically significant only on day 21, whereas the PI from the contralateral ovarian artery depicts an increase that is statistically significant only on day 16. When comparing the PI with both ovarian arteries at each of the four measuring points of the menstrual cycle, the authors found that the PI originating from the ovarian artery related to the ovary carrying the dominant follicle or corpus luteum was significantly lower on days 13, 16 and 21. This reduction was determined by a rise in end-diastolic flow velocity, suggesting that the corpus luteum acts as a low-impedance shunt. The increased blood supply to the functioning corpus luteum is essential for delivery of precursors involved in steroidogenesis and for removal of progesterone. In contrast to an earlier study, no impedance difference was established during the mid-follicular phase (day 7). A significant correlation was documented only on day 21 between the PI from the ovarian artery and uterine artery on the side of the corpus luteum as opposed to the contralateral side during the menstrual cycle, despite the fact that there was a marked reduction in PI from this artery on the side of the ovary carrying the corpus luteum. Comparison of the PI on the side of the ovary bearing the developing corpus luteum suggested reduced downstream impedance or increased blood flow. The authors recorded the highest PI in the uterine arteries on cycle day 16.

De Ziegler and associates[13] conducted a study in young women deprived of ovarian function who received physiological estradiol and progesterone replacement. Their results showed that, in the absence of estrogen production by the ovary, uterine arteries have a high degree of vascular resistance expressed by narrow systolic Doppler flow waveforms and high PI values. This observation differed from the findings made during the early follicular phase of the menstrual cycle, which showed a persistence of blood flow during at least part of the diastolic interval in several women.

This observation is in accordance with the hypothesis that the decrease in vascular resistance observed at the time of ovulation in the menstrual cycle is mediated by estradiol. Because estrogen receptors have been identified in the walls of uterine arteries, it is likely that the effect of estradiol on the uterine Doppler waveform is direct. Therefore, it is reasonable to postulate that the estrogenic effect exerted on the vascular resistance of uterine arteries is directly related to the plasma level of biologically active estrogens reaching the uterine vessels and that a direct dose–effect relationship might exist.

Progesterone administration from days 15 to 28 induced a minor change of uterine artery Doppler waveforms and indicated that progesterone does not interfere markedly with

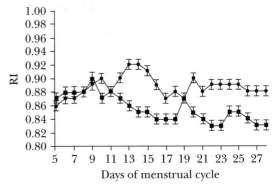

Figure 7 Uterine artery flow velocity in the menstrual cycle, for fertile women (squares) and anovulatory infertile women (circles)

the vasodilatory effect of estradiol on uterine arteries.

Kurjak and associates[5] performed serial measurements of the flow velocity of the uterine and ovarian arteries throughout the menstrual cycle in women attending an infertility clinic, and compared them with measurements from volunteers coming for annual examinations. Uterine flow velocity had an RI of 0.88 ± 0.04 (2 SE) in the proliferative phase, and this started to decrease the day before ovulation. A nadir of 0.84 ± 0.04 (Figure 7) was reached on day 21 and the RI remained at that level for the rest of the cycle. In anovulatory cycles, these changes did not occur. A subgroup of 12 women who lacked end-diastolic flow in the uterine arteries during the secretory phase were identified. Eleven of these women were infertile, eight with primary infertility. Ovarian artery flow velocity was usually detected when the dominant follicle reached 12–15 mm. The RI was 0.54 ± 0.04 and also declined on the day before ovulation. A nadir of 0.44 ± 0.04 was reached 4–5 days later and slowly rose to 0.050 ± 0.04 before menstruation.

Zaidi and co-workers[14] prospectively assessed uterine artery blood flow by transvaginal color and pulsed Doppler ultrasound. Measurements were taken during the periovulatory period. All patients had regular ovulatory menstrual cycles and a mid-luteal serum progesterone level consistent with spontaneous ovulation in the preceding cycle. When the mean follicular diameter was > 16 mm, or day −2 from the estimated day of ovulation was reached, patients were scanned at 6-h intervals at 06.00, 12.00, 18.00 and 24.00 until follicular rupture. The mean uterine artery PI showed a marked daily fluctuation with a nadir occurring most commonly at 06.00. A comparison between the mean PI values at 06.00 and 18.00 showed significantly lower results at 06.00 in both dominant and non-dominant uterine arteries. Mean uterine artery time-averaged maximum velocity showed daily fluctuations with peak values most commonly occurring at 06.00 with the nadir occurring during the afternoon and late evening. There was no temporal relationship between the fluctuations in PI and changes in levels of luteinizing hormone, follicle stimulating hormone, estradiol or progesterone. These observations suggest that there is a circadian rhythm in uterine artery blood flow during the periovulatory period which appears to be independent of hormonal changes.

In spontaneous cycles the mean PI of the radial artery declined from 2.75 measured 2 days before ovulation to 1.19 on the day before ovulation (Figure 8). A significant difference in spiral artery flow velocity (increased flow velocity) marked with PI of 1.13 occurred the day before ovulation in spontaneous cycles (Figure 9).

The same method allows assessment of intraovarian blood flow during the ovarian cycle. Color Doppler facilitates the detection of small vascular areas in the ovarian stroma and follicular rim[5]. Blood flow velocity waveforms from the follicle can be seen when the follicle reaches 10–12 mm in diameter, and these may be a hemodynamic parameter of its growth, maturation and ovulation (Figure 10). The RI is approximately 0.54 ± 0.04 until ovulation approaches[15]. A decline begins 2 days prior to ovulation and the RI reaches its nadir at

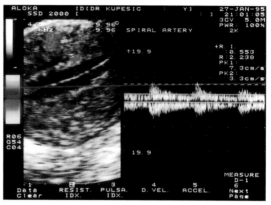

Figure 9 Color signals obtained from the periphery of the multilayered endometrium represent spiral arteries (left). The pulsed Doppler waveform analysis (right) shows low-to-moderate resistance that is characteristic of normal uterine receptivity

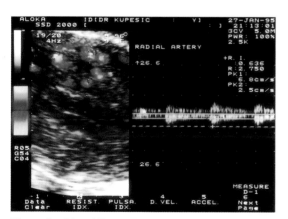

Figure 8 Blood flow velocity waveforms of the radial arteries (right). Note the position of the gate on the left panel (within the myometrium) for sampling flow velocity waveforms. Lower velocity and lower impedence (RI = 0.64) blood flow signals were obtained from the examined vessels

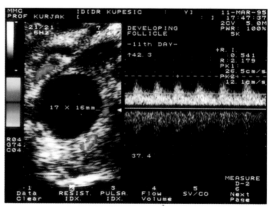

Figure 10 Transvaginal sonogram of the ovary containing a growing follicle. Color Doppler imaging facilitates the detection of a small vascular area surrounding the dominant follicle. The pulsed Doppler waveform analysis of the intraovarian blood flow shows a resistance index of 0.54

ovulation (0.44 ± 0.04). Vascular changes at the time of presumed ovulation show increased vascularity on the inner wall of the follicle and a coincident surge in blood velocity just prior to eruption. Immediately after follicular rupture there is a further dramatic increase in the velocity of blood flow to the early corpus luteum. The RI remains at that level for 4–5 days, then gradually climbs to a level of 0.50 ± 0.04, still lower than that seen in the proliferative phase.

It is hoped that transvaginal color flow and pulsed Doppler ultrasound could be used to optimize the time of recovery of oocytes of the highest quality. Collins and colleagues[16] found that the changes in PI observed from the wall of the dominant follicle and corpus luteum were less marked than the changes in blood velocity. Merce and co-workers[17] obtained Doppler shift waveforms from the parenchyma of the non-dominant ovary and from the parenchyma adjacent to the dominant follicle or corpus luteum in the dominant ovary. Like Kurjak and co-workers[5], they detected a blood flow velocity waveform index in the dominant ovary that was lower during the luteal phase than the follicular phase. Increased resistance to blood flow was observed in the late luteal phase. These blood flow changes reflect changes in vascularization and the function of the corpus luteum. Some experimental studies[17,18] have shown that the blood flow to the dominant ovary decreased dramatically during the late luteal phase of the cycle. The non-dominant ovary[17] presented a slightly higher blood flow velocity waveform index in the luteal than in the follicular phase. Higher blood flow velocity and lower impedance detected in the vessels of the dominant ovary in the late follicular and early luteal phase indicate increased blood flow to the dominant ovary (Figure 11).

The Doppler technique and uptake of radioactive microspheres by the ovary in ewes[19] demonstrated a three- to seven-fold increase of blood flow during the luteal phase. Clearly, in both uterine and ovarian vessels, changes in flow velocity occur before ovulation, implying that these changes are complex and not purely secondary to progesterone action[5]. Undoubtedly, many other vasoactive compounds (e.g. prosta-

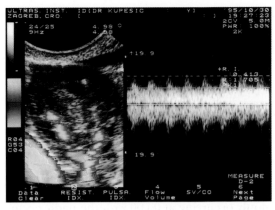

Figure 11 Increased blood flow velocity and decreased resistance index (RI = 0.41) representing typical signs of ovulation and early corpus luteum formation

glandins) are involved in the regulation of the ovarian vasculature.

Kurjak and Kupesic[20] tried to establish the influence of ovarian senescence on uterine and ovarian perfusion. They evaluated 250 patients: 120 healthy fertile controls, 85 postmenopausal patients and 45 postmenopausal patients receiving hormonal replacement therapy. The ovarian artery Doppler measurements in postmenopausal patients showed a significant difference when compared with the ovarian artery on the side containing the dominant follicle or corpus luteum in the healthy fertile group. Absence of intraovarian blood flow velocity waveforms was a normal finding in the postmenopausal group of patients. This was probably owing to a progressive increase in the amount of fibroblasts and connective tissue and a decrease in the concentration of the circulating estrogens. Therefore, any color flow obtained from the postmenopausal ovary should generate a high index of suspicion for abnormal neovascularization and requires detailed pulsed Doppler waveform analysis. Uterine and radial artery flow velocity analyses demonstrated significant positive correlations between the RI values and years of menopause. In patients receiving hormone replacement therapy (HRT) a lowering effect occurred in the RI of the main uterine artery and its intramyometrial branches. Visualization of clear Doppler signals from the spiral arteries was possible in 30% of women who were menopausal for < 5 years. The addition of HRT resulted in higher visualization rates of the spiral arteries and lowered RI values in the uterine arteries. There were changes in the flow velocity patterns of the ovarian, uterine, radial and spiral arteries with age. The fact that the uterine artery RI does not change significantly in the first post-menopausal years strongly supports the thesis that the aging process initially affects the uterus less than the ovary. Therefore, the uterine environment can be manipulated more easily during the menopausal years by proper hormonal stimulation[20].

References

1. Kurjak, A., Kupesic, S., Zalud, I. and Predanic, M. (1995). Transvaginal color Doppler. In Dodson, M. G. (ed.) *Transvaginal Ultrasound*, pp. 325–39. (New York: Churchill Livingstone)
2. Fleischer, A. C., Kepple, D. M. and Entman, S. S. (1991). Transvaginal sonography of uterine disorders. In Timor Tritsch, I. E. and Rottem, S. (eds.) *Transvaginal Sonography*, 2nd edn, pp. 119–30. (New York: Elsevier)
3. Du Bose, T. J., Hill, L. W., Henningan, H. W. Jr *et al.* (1985). Sonography of arcuate uterine blood vessels. *J. Ultrasound Med.*, **4**, 229–33
4. Jurkovic, D., Jauniaux, E., Kurjak, A. *et al.* (1991). Transvaginal color Doppler assessment of the uteroplacental circulation in early pregnancy. *Obstet. Gynecol.*, **77**, 365–9
5. Kurjak, A., Kupesic-Urek, S., Schulman, H. and Zalud, I. (1991). Transvaginal color Doppler in the assessment of ovarian and uterine blood flow in infertile women. *Fertil. Steril.*, **56**, 870–3
6. Goswamy, R. K. and Steptoe, P. C. (1989). Doppler ultrasound studies of the uterine artery in spontaneous ovarian cycles. *Hum. Reprod.*, **3**, 721–3
7. Goswamy, R. K., Wiliams, G. and Steptoe, P. C. (1988). Decreased uterine perfusion a cause of infertility. *Hum. Reprod.*, **3**, 955–8
8. Bourne, T., Jurkovic, D., Waterstone, J., Campbell, S. and Collins, W. P. (1991). Intrafollicular blood flow during human ovulation. *Ultrasound Obstet. Gynecol.*, **1**, 53–7
9. Deutinger, J., Reinthaller, A. and Bernaschek, G. (1989). Transvaginal pulsed Doppler measurement of blood flow velocity in the ovarian arteries during cycle stimulation and after follicle puncture. *Fertil. Steril.*, **51**, 466–70
10. Battaglia, C., Larocca, E., Lanzani, A., Valentini, M. and Genazzani, A. R. (1990). Doppler ultrasound studies of the uterine arteries in spontaneous and IVF cycles. *Gynecol. Endocrinol.*, **4**, 245–50
11. Steer, C. V., Mills, C. V. and Campbell, S. (1991). Vaginal color Doppler assessment on the day of embryo transfer (ET) accurately predicts patients in an *in vitro* fertilization programme with suboptimal uterine perfusion who fail to be pregnant. *Ultrasound Obstet. Gynecol.*, **1**, (Suppl.), 79
12. Scholtes, M. C., Wladimiroff, J. W., van Rijen, H. J. M. and Hop, W. C. J. (1989). Uterine and ovarian flow velocity waveforms in the normal menstrual cycle: a transvaginal Doppler study. *Fertil. Steril.*, **52**, 981–5
13. de Ziegler, D., Bessis, R. and Frydman, R. (1991). Vascular resistance of uterine arteries: physiological effects of estradiol and progesterone. *Fertil. Steril.*, **55**, 775–9
14. Zaidi, J., Jurkovic, D., Campbell, S., Pitroff, R., McGregor, A. and Tan, S. L. (1995). Description of circadian rhythm in uterine artery blood flow during the peri-ovulatory period. *Hum. Reprod.*, **10**, 1642–6
15. Kurjak, A. and Kupesic, S. (1994). Color Doppler velocimetry of the ovary: vaginal approach. In Sabbagha, R. E. (ed.) *Diagnostic Ultrasound Applied to Obstetrics and Gynecology*. (Philadelphia: J.B. Lippincott)
16. Collins, W., Jurkovic, D., Bourne, T., Kurjak, A. and Campbell, S. (1991). Ovarian morphology, endocrine function and intra-follicular blood flow during periovulatory period. *Hum. Reprod.*, **3**, 319–24
17. Merce, L. T., Garces, D., Barco, M. J. and de la Fuente, F. (1992). Intraovarian Doppler velocimetry in ovulatory, dysovulatory and anovulatory cycles. *Ultrasound Obstet. Gynaecol.*, **2**, 197–202
18. Bassett, D. L. (1943). The changes in the vascular pattern of the ovary of the albino rat during the estrous cycle. *Am. J. Anat.*, **73**, 251–91
19. Niswender, G. D., Moore, R. T., Akbar, A. M., Nett, T. M. and Diekman, M. A. (1975). Flow of blood to the ovaries of ewes throughout the estrous cycle. *Biol. Reprod.*, **13**, 381–8
20. Kurjak, A. and Kupesic, S. (1995). Ovarian senescence and its significance on uterine and ovarian perfusion. *Fertil. Steril.*, **64**, 532–7

Color Doppler sonography of benign and malignant adnexal masses: a spectrum of findings

3

A. C. Fleischer

INTRODUCTION

Color Doppler sonography (CDS) provides insight to physiological parameters by its depiction of blood flow (Figure 1). When correlated with the anatomic information provided by transvaginal sonography (TVS), CDS provides clinically important features of adnexal masses.

With the extensive use and expanded clinical experience with CDS of adnexal masses, a better appreciation of the advantages and limitations of this technique has been gained. The data gathered from several studies report an overlap in the impedance values in benign and malig-nant ovarian lesions. There is almost uniform agreement that the blood flow in malignant lesions demonstrates lower impedance and higher velocities than in benign lesions[1,2]. The controversy centers around whether there is a statistically significant threshold value that can be universally applied for differentiation of benign from malignant adnexal masses[3–14]. Part of the controversy is engendered by differences in the patient population, and in the technique and instrumentation used in these studies. Another factor limiting the universal

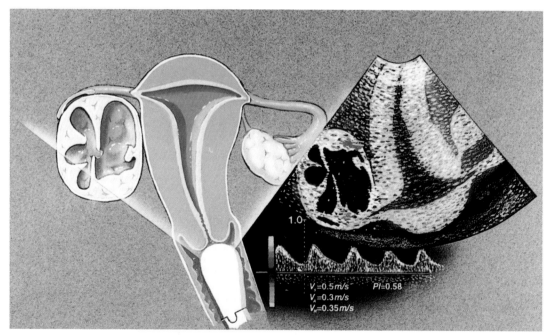

Figure 1 Diagram of transvaginal color Doppler sonography of pelvic masses consisting of real-time image, pulsed range-gated Doppler and spectrum (drawing by Paul Gross, MS)

application of CDS is related to sampling error arising from the choice of which vessels to interrogate; this in turn is related to system sensitivity.

With the acknowledgement of these limitations, CDS is utilized in several leading medical centers and some private offices as an adjunct to transvaginal sonography for the evaluation of adnexal masses, but its use must be correlated with clinical and morphological data.

This chapter presents a critical analysis of the use of CDS for adnexal mass evaluation, with both the potential and the limitations of the technique taken into account. The discussion is based on over 8 years of experience with CDS and its correlation with macro- and microscopic pathology.

CDS PARAMETERS

One of the limitations of CDS is that it samples flow in only a selected vessel rather than displaying data on the overall flow to and within a mass (Figure 2). Accordingly, the impedance within a particular vessel is an indirect reflection of the downstream resistance of the entire vascular network within a mass. This, in turn, is a reflection of the vascular 'tone' provided by the interstitium. Tumor vascularity differs from the orderly and regular vessels seen in a physiological structure such as the corpus luteum by comprising irregularly spaced vessels with numerous arteriovenous shunts, blind-ending vessels and vessels within poor perivascular support and tone. As opposed to non-malignant angiogenesis from the host vasculature by budding from the arteriolar system, tumor vessels typically arise from venous vessels that have relatively poor tone and numerous arteriovenous shunts[15]. Accordingly, the flow in a tumor tends to have lower impedance and increased diastolic flow, areas of relatively high velocity due to focal areas of stenosis, blind ending 'ponds' and shunting.

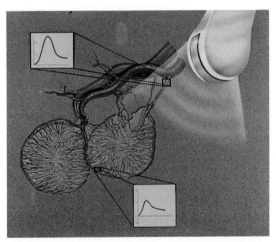

Figure 2 Diagram of vascularity of ovarian mass supplied by radially arranged vessels. Waveforms indicate flow in selected feeding vessels rather than overall flow (drawing by Paul Gross, MS)

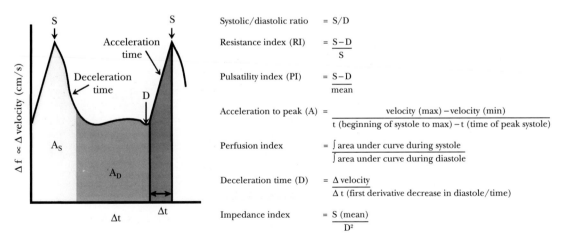

Figure 3 Methods for quantitation of waveform. S, systolic; D, diastolic; Δf, change in frequency; Δvelocity, change in velocity; A_S, area during systole; A_D, area during diastole; Δt, change in time

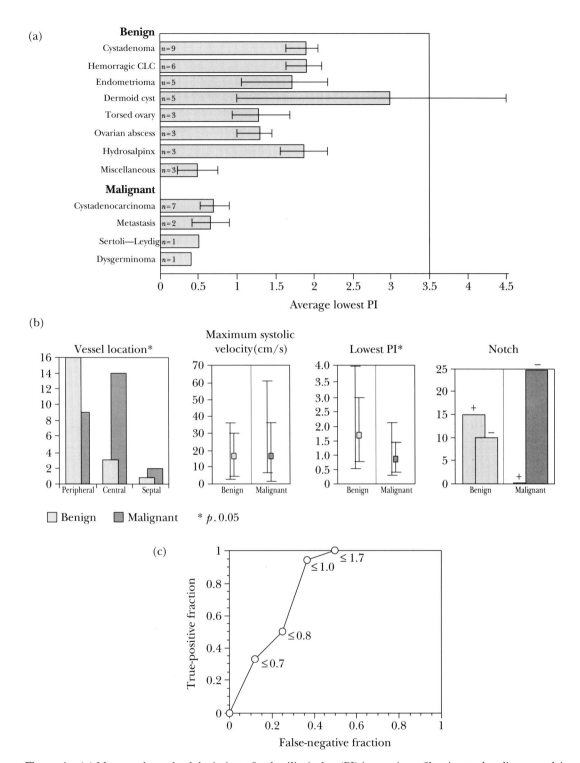

Figure 4 (a) Mean and standard deviation of pulsatility index (PI) in a variety of benign and malignant pelvic masses (from reference 32). CLC, corpus luteum cyst. (b) Mean and range of various parameters in 25 benign and 25 malignant ovarian masses (from reference 25). (c) Receiver operating curve (ROC) with true positive vs. false negative (from reference 17)

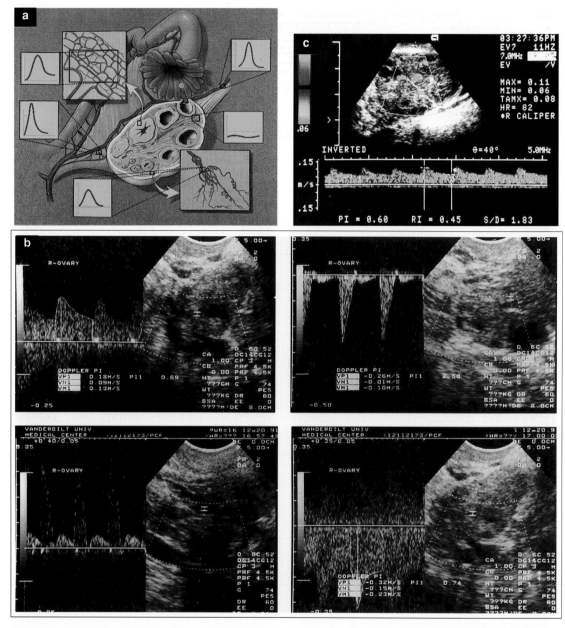

Figure 5 Normal ovarian waveforms. (a) Diagram showing various waveforms around and within the ovary. (b) Color Doppler sonograms showing various impedances within the same ovary (top left); within the wall of the corpus luteum (top right); within a feeding vessel (bottom left); and within a feeding vessel within the wall of the corpus luteum (bottom right). (c) Frequency color Doppler sonography of corpus luteum showing low impedance flow within the wall

Concerning quantification of the spectral waveform, the resistance index (RI) or pulsatility index (PI) seem to be equally accurate in differentiating benign from malignant masses[12]. There are other parameters of the waveform that may be of diagnostic use, such as the acceleration index, which will require further study (Figure 3). With the use of contrast, 'uptake' and 'dwell' times may also be of diagnostic importance when shown on a time–activity curve[16].

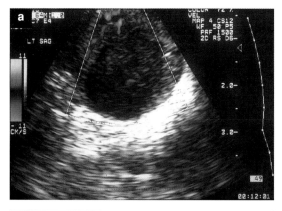

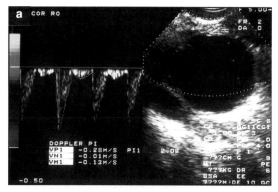

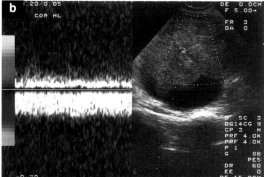

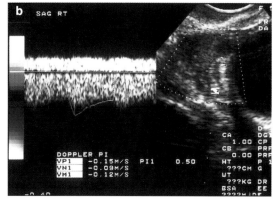

Figure 6 Central vs. peripheral flow. (a) Color Doppler sonography of hemorrhagic corpus luteum with no central flow but peripheral flow. (b) Central flow with low impedance within an irregular solid area of ovarian carcinoma.

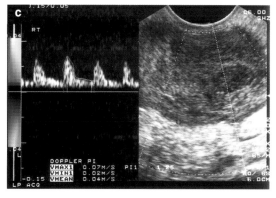

Figure 7 Color Doppler sonography of benign cystic masses. (a) Smooth-walled cyst with high-impedance flow within its wall. (b) Endometrioma before and (c) after stable clot has formed

Clinical studies have reported a spectrum of Doppler parameters in ovarian masses, and since a universal cut-off value may not exist, data may be best expressed in a receiver operating curve (ROC) in which particular values are plotted vs. false-positive and false-negative fractions[17] (Figure 4). The diagnostic accuracy of impedance values in differentiating benign from malignant lesions has ranged from high (over 96%) to poor (less than 40%)[3,18,19]. Statistical analysis of the data from various reports is confounded by non-universal selection of Doppler parameters (resistance vs. pulsatility index), choice of highest, lowest or mean impedance values and selection of vessels to interrogate. Differences in operator variance and system sensitivity contribute to an already confusing analysis of parameters[20].

An excellent analysis[21] of multiple parameters indicates that lower RI (< 0.45; sensitivity 100%, false positives 11.4%) and central tumor location (sensitivity 90%, false-positive site 11.4%) are accurate parameters in differentiating benign from malignant ovarian masses. Others have described sufficiently accurate

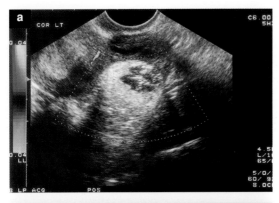

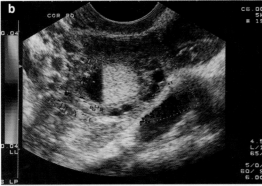

Figure 8 Color Doppler sonography of dermoid cysts. (a) A hypovascular dermoid cyst; and (b) a dermoid cyst with vascularity within its wall

discriminating parameters to be $PI \leq 1.0$ combined with peak systolic maximum velocity of > 12 cm/s to yield a sensitivity of 88.9% and specificity of 88.1%[22]. Presence or absence of a diastolic notch seems to be moderately helpful; this was seen in 89% of benign tumors and in no malignant tumors[23]. Blood vessels were visualized in 95% of malignant tumors and in 70% of benign tumors. In addition, the visualized blood vessels tended to be localized centrally in malignancies (65 vs. 5%). The average number of blood vessels seen in malignancies (six) was statistically significantly higher than in benign lesions (one)[24]. Therefore, multiparameter analysis is recommended as initially described and advocated by this author[25].

BENIGN ADNEXAL MASSES

The vascular network of benign masses consists of orderly branching vessels. The vascular 'tone'

characteristic of these vessels in supported by a muscular media and stroma. Dilatation usually results from several circulating vasogenic substances. It may also occur in inflammatory conditions.

Besides the monthly development of endometrial vascularity, the corpus luteum is one of the few structures that contain a relatively predictable vascular network that develops and regresses[26]. The flow in the wall of the corpus luteum is readily depicted with CDS, particularly amplitude-CDS. The flow within the vessels in the corpus luteum wall is characterized by low impedance and low velocity and is related to its physiological function (Figure 5). Thin-walled corpora lutea tend to have less apparent flow than thick-walled corpora lutea[26]. Hemorrhagic lesions display a central flow, as opposed to solid lesions, which contain vascularized tissue (Figure 6).

The most common adnexal lesions to contain internal hemorrhage are hemorrhagic corpus luteum and endometrioma. Various amounts of impedance can be seen within the wall of the corpus luteum, depending on its developmental stage. Similarly, the blood flow within the endometrium can also vary, with the lowest impedance coinciding with menses (Figure 7).

Dermoid cysts typically exhibit flow within their walls and have a spectrum of waveforms. Centrally located flow may suggest struma ovarii, which represents endocrinologically functional tissue within the mass (Figure 8).

Benign epithelial tumors of the ovary may exhibit flow within the wall and/or septae. Low-impedance flow can be observed within the septae even in benign lesions. These vessels usually have deficient muscular media, but the septae in which they are contained is typically thin and regular (Figure 9). High impedance or no flow can be seen in some benign or malignant lesions due to torsion. Intercurrent vascular disease may also affect flow to and within adnexal lesions.

MALIGNANT ADNEXAL MASSES

Based on morphology, malignancy should be suspected when a mass contains irregular

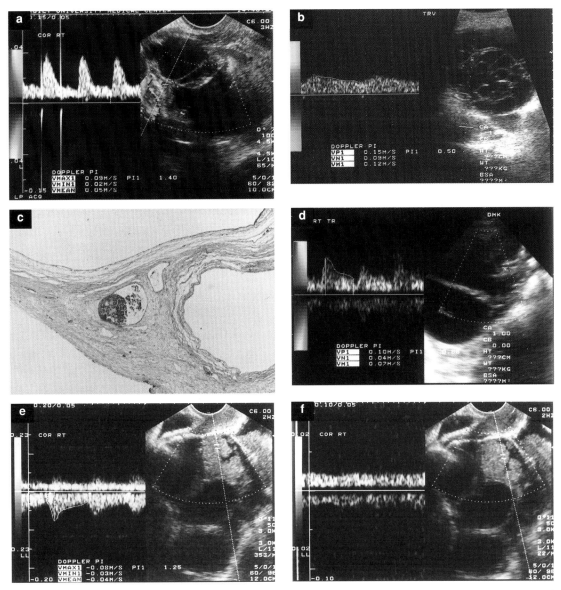

Figure 9 Benign and malignant septated masses. (a) High impedance flow (PI = 1.4) in a benign septated mass; (b) septated mass with low impedance within a septal vessel; (c) low-power photomicrograph showing abnormal vessel within septum of mass shown in (b). This was a borderline ovarian cancer; (d) malignant ovarian tumor showing low impedance within a papillary excrescence. Intermediate impedance arterial (e) and venous (f) flow within a solid area of an ovarian cancer, appearing as a septated mass with a thick and irregular wall

septae, papillary excrescences and solid areas. CDS provides adjunctive means to confirm the suspicion of malignancy. In most cases, the blood flow within malignancies exhibits low impedance and high velocity in morphologically suspicious areas (Figure 10).

The CDS findings that are observed will depend on several intrinsic factors (related to the mass itself) and extrinsic factors (related to technique and equipment). The presence and extent of tumor vascularization is related to the stage of growth at which it is examined. In the

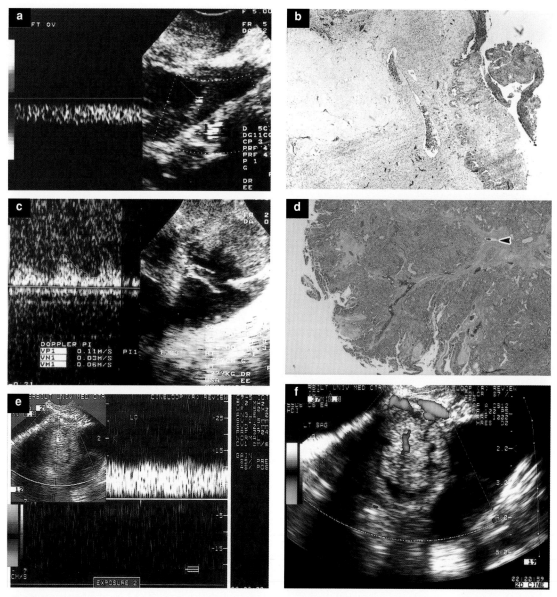

Figure 10 Ovarian cancer. (a) Venous-like waveform arising from irregular wall. (b) Low-power photomicrograph, showing tumor vessel within this ovarian cancer seen in (a). (c) Frequency-color Doppler sonography of papillary cystadenocarcinoma extending into distended left tube. (d) Photomicrograph of (c) showing tumor vessels (arrowhead). (e) Frequency-color Doppler sonography showing low-impedance flow within papillary excrescence. (f) Amplitude color Doppler sonography showing vessel within papillary excrescence. This was a papillary serous cystadenocarcinoma

early and rapid stage of growth, extensive tumor vascularization with its typical low-impedance, high-velocity flow is usually observed. However, once tumor growth is beyond its peak, tumor necrosis may result in areas of variable impedance[27]. The morphology of the tumor can also

influence the CDS findings. The overlap of impedance can be observed in solid lesions more than in separated lesions[28].

In general, malignancies exhibit morphological abnormality and low-impedance, high-velocity flow. Occasionally, malignancy can be suspected initially on the CDS features alone. It should be remembered that the diagnostic use of CDS must be integrated with the clinical features. Adding Doppler sonography to transvaginal sonography provides specificity and positive prediction values higher than with CDS alone. In one report, the specificity increased from 82% to 97% ($p < 0.001$) and the positive predictive value increased from 63% to 91%[29]. Further investigation concerning the optimization or weighting of CDS parameters would seem to be potentially useful[30].

SUMMARY

The differentiation of benign from malignant ovarian masses based on CDS requires consideration of technical and intrinsic factors. Although a specific cut-off value may not exist, multiparameter analysis combined with clinical assessment can provide clinically pertinent data concerning the likelihood of malignancy in these masses. Further technical refinements in CDS quantification of flow, such as described in implanted tumors, may improve diagnostic accuracy and allow for serial evaluation[31].

References

1. Kurjak, A. and Predanic, M. (1992). New scoring system for prediction of ovarian malignancy based on transvaginal color Doppler sonography. *J. Ultrasound Med.*, **11**, 631–8
2. Fleischer, A. C., Cullinan, J. A., Peery, C. V. and Jones, H. W. (1996). Early detection of ovarian carcinoma with transvaginal color Doppler ultrasonography. Am. J. Obstet. Gyencol., 174, 101–6
3. Tekay, A. and Jouppila, P. (1992). Validity of pulsatility and resistance indices in classification of adnexal tumors with transvaginal color Doppler ultrasound. *Ultrasound Obstet. Gynecol.*, **2**, 338–44
4. Bromley, B., Goodman, H. and Benacerraf, B. R. (1994). Comparison between sonographic morphology and Doppler waveform for the diagnosis of ovarian malignancy. *Obstet. Gynecol.*, **83**, 434–7
5. Salem, S., White, L. M. and Lai, J. (1994). Doppler sonography of adnexal masses: the predictive value of the pulsatility index in benign and malignant disease. *Am. J. Roentgenol.*, **163**, 1147–50
6. Hamper, U. M., Sheth, S., Abbas, F. M., Rosenshein, N. B., Aronson, D. and Kurman, R. J. (1993). Transvaginal color Doppler sonography of adnexal masses: differences in blood flow impedance in benign and malignant lesions. *Am. J. Roentgenol.*, **160**, 1225–8
7. Valentin, L., Sladkevicius, P. and Marsàl, K. (1994). Limited contribution of Doppler velocimetry to the differential diagnosis of extrauterine pelvic tumors. *Obstet. Gynecol.*, **83**, 425–9
8. Timor-Tritsch, I. E., Lerner, J. P., Monteagudo, A. and Santos, R. (1993). Transvaginal ultrasonographic characterization of ovarian masses by means of color flow-directed Doppler measurements and a morphologic scoring system. *Am. J. Obstet. Gynecol.*, **168**, 909–13
9. Stein, S. M., Laifer-Narin, S., Johnson, M. B., Roman, L. D., Muderspach, L. I., Tyszka, J. M. and Ralls, P. W. (1995). Differentiation of benign and malignant adnexal masses: relative value of gray-scale, color Doppler, and spectral Doppler sonography. *Am. J. Roentgenol.*, **164**, 381–6
10. Lin, P. Y., Lai, J. I., Wu, C. C., Lee, C. N., Chen, C. A., Hsieh, C. Y. and Hsieh, F. J. (1993). Color Doppler ultrasound in the assessment of ovarian neoplasms. *J. Med. Ultrasound*, **1**, 172–6
11. Tepper, R., Lerner-Geva, L., Altaras, M. M., Goldberger, S., Ben-Baruch, G., Markov, S., Cohen, I. and Byeth, Y. (1995). Transvaginal color flow imaging in the diagnosis of ovarian tumors. *J. Ultrasound Med.*, **14**, 731–4
12. Carter, J., Saltzman, A., Hartenbach, E., Fowler, J., Carson, L. and Twiggs, L. B. (1994). Flow characteristics in benign and malignant gynecologic tumors using transvaginal color flow Doppler. *Obstet. Gynecol.*, **83**, 125–30
13. Weiner, Z., Thaler, I., Beck, D., Rottem, S., Deutsch, M. and Brandes, J. M. (1992). Differentiating malignant from benign ovarian tumors with transvaginal color flow imaging. *Obstet. Gynecol.*, **79**, 159–62
14. Kawai, M., Kano, T., Kikkawa, F., Maeda, O., Oguchi, H. and Tomoda, Y. (1992). Transvaginal Doppler ultrasound with color flow imaging in the diagnosis of ovarian cancer. *Obstet. Gynecol.*, **79**, 163–7
15. Schoenfeld, A., Levavi, H., Tepper, R. *et al.* (1994). Assessment of tumor-indicated angiogenesis by three-dimensional display: confusing

Doppler signals in ovarian cancer screening? (Letter to editor). *Ultrasound Obstet. Gynecol.*, **4**, 516

16. Cosgrove, D. (1997). Evaluation of tumors using echo-enhancing agents. In Goldberg, B. (ed.) *Ultrasonic Contrast Agents.* (London: Martin Dunitz)

17. Carter, J. R., Lau, M., Fowler, J. M., Carlson, J. W., Carson, L. F. and Twiggs, L. B. (1995). Blood flow characteristics of ovarian tumors: implications for ovarian cancer screening. *Am. J. Obstet. Gynecol.*, **172**, 901–7

18. Kurjak, A. and Kupesic, S. (1995). Transvaginal color Doppler and pelvic tumor vascularity: lessons learned and future challenges. *Ultrasound Obstet. Gynecol.*, **6**, 145–59

19. Levine, D., Feldstein, V. A., Babcook, C. J. and Filly, R. A. (1994). Sonography of ovarian masses: poor sensitivity of resistive index for indentifying malignant lesions. *Am. J. Roentgenol.*, **162**, 1355–9

20. Pellerito, J. S., Troiano, R. N., Quedens-Case, C. and Taylor, K. J. W. (1995). Common pitfalls of endovaginal color Doppler flow imaging. *Radio-Graphics*, **15**, 37–47

21. Alcázar, J. L., Ruiz-Perez, M. L. and Errasti, T. (1996). Transvaginal color Doppler sonography in adnexal masses: which parameter performs best? *Ultrasound Obstet. Gynecol.*, **8**, 114–19

22. Tailor, A., Jurkovic, D., Bourne, T. H., Natucci, M., Collins, W. P. and Campbell, S. (1996). A comparison of intratumoral indices of blood flow velocity and impedance for the diagnosis of ovarian cancer. *Ultrasound Med. Biol.*, **22**, 837–43

23. Maly, Z., Riss, P. and Deutinger, J. (1995). Localization of blood vessels and qualitative assessment of blood flow in ovarian tumors. *Obstet. Gynecol.*, **85**, 33–6

24. Wu, C. C., Lee, C. N., Chen, T. M., Lai, J. I., Hsieh, C. Y. and Hsieh, F. J. (1994). Factors con-tributing to the accuracy in diagnosing ovarian malignancy by color Doppler ultrasound. *Obstet. Gynecol.*, **84**, 1–4

25. Fleischer, A. C., Rodgers, W. H., Kepple, D. M., Williams, L. L. and Jones, H. W. (1993). Color Doppler sonography of ovarian masses: a multi-parameter analysis. *J. Ultrasound Med.*, **12**, 41–8

26. Parsons, A. (1994). Ultrasound of the human corpus luteum. *Ultrasound Q.*, **12**, 127–66

27. Fleischer, A., Cullivan, J., Jones, H., Peery, C. *et al.* (1995). Serial assessment of adnexal masses with transvaginal color Doppler sonography. *Ultrasound Med. Biol.*, **21**, 435–41

28. Sladkevicius, P., Valentin, L. and Marsál, K. (1995). Transvaginal Doppler examination for the differential diagnosis of solid pelvic tumors. *J. Ultrasound Med.*, **14**, 377–80

29. Buy, J. N., Ghossain, M. A., Hugol, D., Hassen, K., Sciot, C., Truc, J. B., Poitout, P. and Vadrot, D. (1996). Characterization of adnexal masses: combination of color Doppler and conventional sonography compared with spectral Doppler analysis alone and conventional sonography alone. *Am. J. Roentgenol.*, **166**, 385–93

30. Brown, D. L., Frates, M. C., Laing, F. C., DiSalvo, D. N., Doubilet, P. M., Benson, C. B., Waitzkin, E. D. and Muto, M. G. (1994). Ovarian masses: can benign and malignant lesions be differen-tiated with color and pulsed Doppler US? *Radiology*, **190**, 333–6

31. Meyerowitz, C. B., Fleischer, A. C., Pickens, D. R., Thurman, G. B., Borowsky, A. D., Thirsk, G. and Hellerqvist, C. G. (1996). Quantification of tumor vascularity and flow with amplitude color Doppler sonography in an experimental model: preliminary results. *J. Ultrasound Med.*, **15**, 827–33

32. Fleischer, A. C., Rodgers, W. and Rao, B. (1991). Assessment of ovarian tumor vascularity with transvaginal color Doppler sonography. *J. Ultrasound Med.*, **10**, 563

Benign adnexal masses assessed by color and pulsed Doppler

4

A. Kurjak and S. Kupesic

Ovarian lesions are a cause of great concern, because of their malignant potential and the limited ability to distinguish accurately between benign and malignant neoplasms prior to surgery. This is particularly true for bizarre structures such as dermoid cysts, huge endometriomas, complex corpus luteum cysts and cystadenomas.

The normal ovary is relatively easy to detect by transvaginal sonography. The first ultrasonographic image of a normal ovary was reported by Kratochwil and colleagues[1]. Its appearance is characterized by the presence of the follicles or the corpus luteum. The ovary is usually located above and medial to the hypogastric vein. During examination, the normal-sized ovary may change its location in the pelvis, because of its mobility, and this may also occur in cases of chronic inflammatory changes, owing to adhesions.

The vascularization of normally functioning ovaries can be detected by color Doppler sonography. Evaluation of follicular development by ultrasound is a well-established procedure in infertility treatment. Blood flow may be clearly visualized at the edge of the developing follicle. The appearance of the corpus luteum is well marked, and color flow is more easily obtainable from the ovarian tissue during the luteal phase. An abundant color pattern, displayed over the ovarian B-mode image, emphasizes the active corpus luteum even when the corpus luteum is not sonographically visible.

In polycystic ovarian disease, the ovaries become enlarged and the ovarian shape becomes more spherical, with the ovarian diameter exceeding the anteroposterior diameter of the uterine fundus. Polycystic ovaries are usually twice the normal size, but approximately one-third of patients may have normal-sized ovaries. These ovaries are characterized by the presence of multiple small cystic structures (< 10 mm) and an increase in volume of the ovarian stroma[2,3]. Cysts may be distributed predominantly around the periphery or scattered throughout the stroma. Increased stroma is the most important diagnostic sign that helps to differentiate polycystic from multifollicular ovaries, which are a temporary feature of normal pubertal development and can be seen in cases of weight loss amenorrhea[4]. Polycystic-appearing ovaries may be visualized in patients who have been taking oral contraceptive pills, in some endocrinological disorders, in pituitary adenoma and in virilizing ovarian and adrenal tumors. The intraovarian vascularity in cases of polycystic ovaries is localized within the ovarian stroma (Figure 1a) and the mean resistance index (RI) is 0.54 without cyclic changes (Figure 1b).

Enlarged ovaries can be divided into three categories: cystic lesions, cystic–solid ovarian masses and solid ovarian neoplasms.

The commonest type of cystic adnexal lesions (Table 1) are *functional ovarian cysts*. These are easily recognizable cystic structures with smooth thin walls and clear fluid contents; they are usually unilateral[5]. These cysts originate from unruptured follicles and are usually smaller than 10 cm. Normal ovarian tissue can be seen along part of the cyst wall. Pericystic vascularization shows moderate resistance to blood flow (RI = 0.52 ± 0.06).

The *corpus luteum cyst* has numerous appearances when imaged transvaginally. Internal echoes created by the retracting clot make it difficult to distinguish this from other benign and malignant ovarian tumors. The dimension of a persistent corpus luteum may exceed 10 cm and its inner structure may appear liquid, solid, or both; it may contain septa (Figure 2a) or even

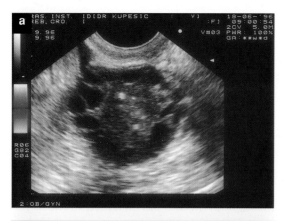

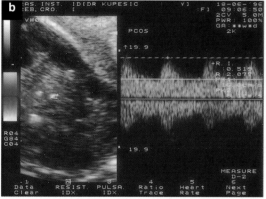

Figure 1 Transvaginal scans of a polycystic ovary. A large number of small cystic structures (a) are crowded together and stand out from the surface of the enlarged ovarian stroma. Pulsed Doppler waveform analysis (b) obtained from the stroma demonstrates moderate impedance to flow (RI = 0.52)

papillae. Unfortunately, the corpus luteum also shows rich angiogenic activity with abundant low-resistance vessels (RI = 0.46 ± 0.08) (Figure 2b). Therefore, the main guideline for avoiding an incorrect diagnosis of this 'great imitator' is to scan premenopausal patients at the beginning of the menstrual cycle[6].

The commonest ovarian epithelial tumors are *serous and mucinous cystadenomas*. These have a specific ultrasonic appearance expressed mostly as multilocular cysts. They are usually large and contain clear fluid with a very low echogenic pattern with linear internal septa that are more pronounced in the mucinous type. The main characteristic is the presence of thin septations, less than 3 mm in diameter. Papillary projections can also be visualized in both serous and mucinous cystadenomas (Figure 3a). The vascular location and type of angiogenesis are important parameters to determine in reducing the overlap with malignant tumors. A moderate RI (0.50 ± 0.08) is usually obtained from peripheral and regularly separated vessels. The vessel type and elevated vascular resistance indicate the benign nature of the lesion (Figure 3b). Vessels displayed within septae are reported to have a slightly lower RI (0.48 ± 0.04).

Paraovarian cysts develop from Gartner's duct and have the same appearance as functional cysts. Only occasionally are they distinguishable from them. Paraovarian cysts can measure as little as 2–3 cm, but more often grow to be quite large[7,8]. A thin and smooth wall, lack of septation within the cystic cavity, sonolucent fluid and preserved ovarian tissue are indicators of a

Table 1 Transvaginal color Doppler in the assessment of benign adnexal masses

Histopathology	n	Color flow		Resistance index	SD
		n	%		
Functional cyst					
follicular cyst	92	84	91.3	0.52	0.06
corpus luteum	104	104	100	0.46	0.08
Dermoid cyst	32	9	28.1	0.48	0.10
Cystadenoma	56	50	89.3	0.50	0.08
Fibroma	7	5	71.4	0.46	0.04
Theca–granulosa cell tumor	2	2	100	0.60	0.04
Brenner's tumor	4	3	75	0.50	0.08
Endometriosis	152	137	90.1	0.49	0.11
Pelvic inflammatory disease	184	134	72.8	0.54	0.12
All cases	633	528	83.4	0.50	0.08

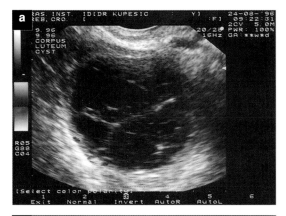

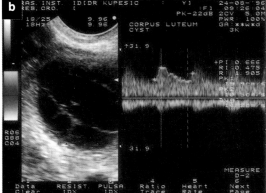

Figure 2 Transvaginal sonograms of a corpus luteum cyst. Color Doppler imaging (a) demonstrates pericystic flow. (b) A high blood flow velocity and low resistance index (RI = 0.47) represent the typical flow pattern of a corpus luteum cyst

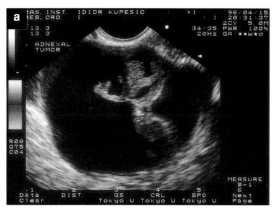

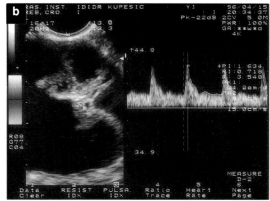

Figure 3 Transvaginal sonograms of a complex tumor. (a) The interior is divided into a number of thick septa, papillary protrusions or loculi containing a clear viscid fluid. Septal neovascular signals are visualized by color Doppler. (b) Doppler measurement (in the same patient) shows high vascular impedance (RI = 0.72) indicating the benign nature of the tumor. Serous cystadenoma was confirmed by histopathology

paraovarian cyst. These lesions usually do not reveal increased vascularity

Dense echogenic contents of the cysts are usually correlated with *mucinous cystadenomas* or *endometriomas*. A homogeneous 'carpet' of low-level echoes in a cystic pelvic mass is a common finding in ovarian endometrioma. Kupfer and associates[9] detected this pattern in 82% of studied cases. One or several sites may be involved in a multilocular mass, or this may be seen dispersed throughout the lesions. Low-level echoes probably represent degraded blood products associated with cyclic changes occurring during the menstrual cycle. The presence of a geographically irregular hyperechoic region in-

ternally can be associated with a more acute phase of hemorrhage. There is usually a well-demarcated separation between the endometrial cyst wall and the normal adjacent ovarian stroma. The most prominent area of vascularization is at the level of the ovarian hilus (Figure 4a), and this has been observed in 78.6% of endometriomas[10]. The RI values measured from this location are usually above 0.45. A recent Doppler study[10] demonstrated a different vascular pattern obtained from endometrioma in proliferative and secretory phases of the menstrual cycle. Furthermore, in the initial stage, extensive angiogenic activity important for further outgrowth and progression of the endometrial

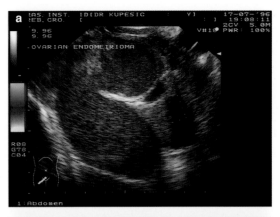

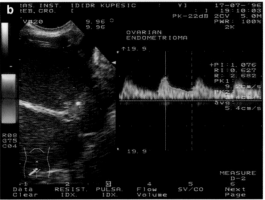

Figure 4 Ovarian endometrioma. (a) Note the homogeneous high-level internal echoes and prominent vascularization at the level of the ovarian hilus. (b) Pulsed Doppler analysis (right), in the same patient, shows moderate impedance (RI = 0.63)

implant demonstrates low to moderate impedance to blood flow (RI = 0.44 ± 0.06). The collagen layer, extent of fibrosis and focal hemorrhage have been reported to alter the vascularity and diffusion of the nutrients into the endometrioma. Higher impedance values (RI = 0.51 ± 0.09) were typical for advanced stages (Figure 4b). Additionally, increased pressure caused by accumulation of 'chocolate' fluid may change the vascularity; this results in an impaired response to both endogenous and exogenous hormones.

Approximately 15% of all ovarian tumors are of the germ cell variety, and of these, over 96% are benign *cystic teratomas*[11-13]. The majority of such lesions occur as asymptomatic adnexal masses. However, the incidence of torsions of

dermoid cysts is as high as 16%[12-14], and occasionally the tumor may rupture, producing acute peritonitis[12,14]. The incidence of malignancy associated with ovarian teratomas is 1–3%[11-14]. In the review by Caruso and associates[12] of 305 consecutive ovarian teratomas from a single unit, the average age for patients with malignant components was 60.8 years.

Several authors retrospectively investigated the various echo patterns of cystic teratomas that may distinguish them from other ovarian lesions. A specific ultrasonic appearance has been described by Quinn and colleagues[15] and reported as the Rokitansky protuberance[6]. Other sonographic signs included dermoid plug[15], 'tip of the iceberg'[16], fat fluid level[17], cysts with a pearl-gray appearance[18] and dermoid mesh representing matted hair[19]. In addition, prominent acoustic shadowing observed behind the echogenic focus accompanied all types of echo presentation. Evidently, a bizarre structure and the absence of any pathognomonic pattern aggravate correct diagnosis of ovarian dermoids.

Therefore, Cohen and Sabbagha[20] proposed additional sonographic criteria for diagnosis, including echogenic tubercle associated with a cystic echo pattern, thin echogenic band-like echoes and/or a dense echo pattern with or without a cystic component (Figure 5a). Unfortunately, malignant tumors sometimes show the same or similar appearance. Even an experienced ultrasonographer using sensitive equipment cannot escape the occasional misinterpretation between a benign adnexal lesion and a malignant one if using morphology alone. Indeed, overlapping with ovarian endometriosis is possible owing to its complex texture and thick walls, and the solid echogenic appearance of hemorrhagic clots within the cystic cavity. Pelvic inflammatory disease (PID) is another entity that may mimic a wide variety of findings, such as dermoids, endometriosis, and sometimes even malignancy. Accurate and reliable differentiation may influence management, because malignant lesions require an aggressive therapeutic approach, including extensive surgical interventions, whereas endometriomas, dermoids and pelvic inflammation may be

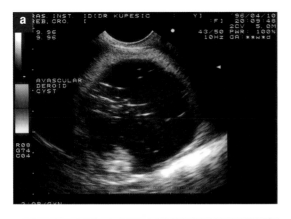

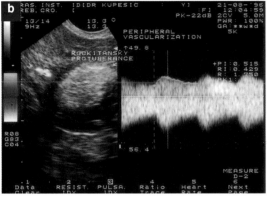

Figure 5 Transvaginal sonogram of a dermoid cyst (a). Note the echogenicity of the solid tumor part and bizarre intracystic echoes. Superimposed color Doppler (b) demonstrates regularly separated vessels on the periphery of the Rokitansky protuberance. Low resistance flow (RI = 0.43) is indicative of inflammatory changes within the dermoid

treated non-invasively or by means of minimally invasive surgery.

An additional parameter that can be used for discrimination between malignant and benign lesions is vascularity. Malignant ovarian tumors are reported to contain a dilated, saccular and randomly dispersed vasculature with typical tortuous course, and a relative paucity of smooth muscle in the media of these vessels[6]. Tumoral neovascularity is marked with arteriovenous communications and tumoral lakes. These vessels exhibit diminished resistance to flow that is demonstrated by high velocity and low resistance. However, increased vascularity has also been demonstrated in some benign entities, such as tubo-ovarian abscesses[21], ovarian endo-

metriomas[10], active hemorrhagic luteal cysts and dermoid cysts with inflammatory changes. All these masses have in common enlarged vascular spaces which can simulate the flow pattern obtained in some malignant ovarian tumors.

During the last 7 years numerous studies have used transvaginal ultrasonography with color flow imaging as a secondary test to reduce the false-positive rate of ultrasound-based screening for ovarian malignancy[6,10,21–30].

Jain[31] analyzed 50 adnexal masses among which five were dermoid cysts. One false-negative case on transvaginal sonography was diagnosed at histopathology as being a borderline malignant dermoid tumor. The same tumor had a high-resistance flow pattern suggestive of a benign diagnosis. Furthermore, one dermoid had low-resistance flow (RI < 0.40) and was wrongly interpreted as ovarian carcinoma.

In a recent study, Hata and co-workers[32] analyzed 63 patients with ovarian tumors, 14 of which were dermoids. Transvaginal sonography identified the features suggestive of malignancy in seven of them. Color Doppler imaging indicated ovarian malignancy in four cystic teratomas with the use of an unusually high cut-off value of 0.72 for the RI.

Weiner and colleagues[33] analyzed 62 women with adnexal tumors. In ten patients dermoid cyst was the definitive diagnosis at histopathology. In three patients with cystic teratoma, B-mode findings were suspicious of malignancy. In two of them, CA 125 levels were over 35 IU/ml. However, transvaginal color and pulsed Doppler analysis demonstrated high impedance values (pulsatility index (PI) > 1.0) in all of them. Color Doppler helped to avoid false positives.

Fleischer and co-workers[34] reported the results of combined transvaginal and color Doppler analysis on 96 adnexal masses. Using transvaginal sonography alone, they were able correctly to differentiate four out of six dermoids. However, when transvaginal ultrasound was combined with color imaging, correct diagnosis was obtained in all six cases.

Campbell and co-workers[35] evaluated the use of transvaginal ultrasonography with color flow imaging as a second-stage test in a screening program for early familial ovarian cancer. The most common source of false positives were endometriosis (four out of nine) and cystic teratoma (two out of nine).

Timor-Tritsch and associates[25] correlated ultrasonographic and histopathological findings of 115 adnexal masses. They correctly diagnosed nine dermoid cysts, applying both morphological score and color flow-directed Doppler measurements. Resistance and pulsatility indices were > 0.46 and > 0.62, respectively.

Our study[24] showed that a small proportion of cystic teratomas (27%) demonstrated increased vascularity. Those vascularized teratomas had resistance to blood flow above our own cut-off value proposed for screening for ovarian carcinoma.

Low to moderate impedance blood flow signals (RI = 0.42–0.72) obtained from a cystic teratoma were derived from an area of actively dividing cells and an area of inflammation, as identified by histopathology (Figure 5b). In contrast to these findings, established stagnant masses did not demonstrate any vascularity.

In the third group of ovarian enlargements there are solid ovarian tumors. The commonest benign solid ovarian tumors are *ovarian fibromas* (and some dermoids). They are usually round in shape with a well-delineated hyperechogenic appearance (Figure 6a). Intratumoral vascularization (centrally or peripherally located) is rarely seen. In vascularized lesions, vessels with high impedance to blood flow may regularly be detected (Figure 6b).

Pelvic inflammatory disease is a serious complication of sexually transmitted microbial infection that can cause permanent damage to the upper reproductive tract. About 30% of infertility cases and 50% of ectopic pregnancies are attributed to previous PID. Adnexal findings include enlarged ovaries, an adnexal tubular anechoic structure or a complex adnexal mass. It is possible to visualize a complex adnexal mass with septate sonographic appearance and irregular external margins, scattered internal echoes and fluid debris levels. Such a finding suggests the presence of a tubo-ovarian abscess. As this may resemble a variety of benign and malignant adnexal conditions (tubal abortions,

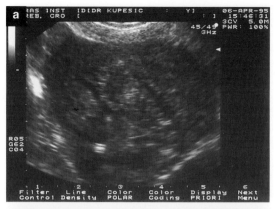

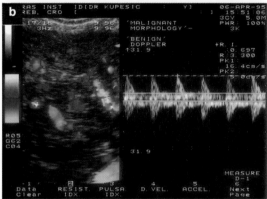

Figure 6 Transvaginal scan (a) demonstrating a case of solid ovarian tumor. Pulsed Doppler sonogram (b) shows reduced diastolic flow (RI = 0.70). Increased vascular resistance is indicative of pre-existing vessels with a normal wall structure. Ovarian fibroma was confirmed by histopathology

hematosalpinx and ovarian tumors), rational combining of morphological and Doppler findings with clinical and biochemical ones enables the correct diagnosis to be reached.

In acute pelvic inflammation the progressive vasodilatation is mediated by local products of inflammation which cause a decrease in RI (0.53 ± 0.09)[21]. Subsequent increased fluid collection within the tubes influences the blood flow characteristics by compressing the vessel walls. As the process advances, the proliferation of the fibroblasts and scar formation leads toward reduction of the local blood flow, demonstrated by the progressive increase in RI (0.71 ± 0.07). Therefore, Doppler studies may be particularly useful in assessing the chronic stage of PID, which may present

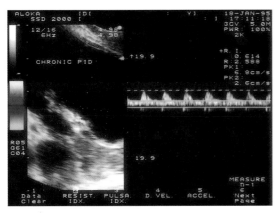

Figure 7 Chronic pelvic inflammation. Color flow is visualized within the walls of the Fallopian tube and pseudopapillary protrusions (left). Pulsed Doppler (right) shows moderate resistance to flow (RI = 0.61), indicating the benign nature of the lesion

pseudopapillomatous structures that morphologically suggest malignancy (Figure 7). The absence of blood flow, typical for this stage, helps to differentiate it from adnexal malignancy[21].

Until the introduction of transvaginal color and pulsed Doppler, morphological criteria were the only parameters taken into consideration[36]. Careful search through the Doppler literature suggests that the high predictive value of transvaginal color Doppler determines the appropriate treatment option: follow-up, minimally invasive surgery or laparotomy.

Scoring systems reported from our department have effectively decreased the rate of both false-positive and false-negative results in differentiation of ovarian lesions[10,21,24]. In comparison of the scoring systems for endometriosis (Table 2) and dermoid cysts (Table 3), some similarities are found. These include reproductive age, positive serial sonography, thick walls and the existence of echogenic contents. However, there are important differences, such as localization (retrouterine in endometriosis vs. lateral with dermoid cysts), bilaterality (in endometriosis vs. unilaterality in dermoids) and the presence and type of vascularization. Ovarian endometriomata were vascularized in 88.3%, mostly at the level of the ovarian hilus, while cystic teratomata were predominantly avascularized (72.6%).

Table 2 Scoring system for endometriosis based on transvaginal color and pulsed Doppler sonography

	Score
Reproductive age	2
Chronic pain (premenstrual or menstrual)	1
Infertility	1
B-mode	
Position (medial, retrouterine)	2
Bilaterality	1
Serial sonography positive	2
Thick walls	2
Homogeneous echogenicity	2
Clear demarcation from the ovary	1
Transvaginal color Doppler	
Vascularization	2
Pericystic/hilar location	2
Regularly separated vessels	2
Existence of notching	1
RI < 0.40 (menstrual phase)	2
RI = 0.41 to 0.60 (late follicular/corpus luteum phase)	2
CA 125 (> 35 IU/ml)	2

Table 3 Scoring system for dermoid cysts based on transvaginal color and pulsed Doppler

	Score
Reproductive age	2
B-mode	
Laterally positioned	2
Unilateral	1
Serial sonography positive	2
Thick walls	2
Thin echogenic band-like echoes	2
Echogenic tubercle within the ovary	2
Fat fluid level	2
Accompanying acoustic shadow	2
No clear demarcation from the ovary	2
Color Doppler analysis	
No vascularization	2

Obviously, there is still a possibility for confusing an endometrioma and a dermoid cyst, but there is a high probability for an experienced sonographer not to confuse these with ovarian malignancy.

In our experience, transvaginal color and pulsed Doppler may serve as a reliable and noninvasive preoperative test. Its routine application has increased the number of laparoscopic procedures during recent years in our department, and no malignancy has been misinterpreted.

Since most of our patients suffering from benign ovarian lesions are of reproductive age, changing the approach to minimally invasive surgery seems to help the preservation of their reproductive potential. Considering that malignancy is very uncommon in this age group[11-13], we believe that expert laparoscopic management in selected cases, with careful technique to minimize the chance of spillage of cystic contents, is a safe and beneficial alternative to laparotomy.

References

1. Kratochwill, A., Urban, G. and Friedrich, F. (1972). Ultrasonic tomography of the ovaries. *Ann. Chir. Gynecol.*, **61**, 211–14
2. Battaglia, C., Artini, P. G., Genazzani, A. D., Sgherzi, M. R., Salvatori, M., Giulini, S. and Volpe, A. (1996). Color Doppler analysis in lean and obese women with polycystic ovary syndrome. *Ultrasound Obstet. Gynecol.*, **7**, 342–6
3. Kupesic, S., Kurjak, A. and Stilinovic, K. (1994). The assessment of female infertility. In Kurjak, A. (ed.) *An Atlas of Transvaginal Color Doppler*, pp. 171–97. (Carnforth, UK: Parthenon Publishing)
4. Obbrai, M., Lyrich, S. S., Holder, G., Jackson, R., Tang, L. and Butt, W. E. (1990). Hormonal studies on women with polycystic ovaries diagnosed by ultrasound. *Clin. Endocrinol.*, **32**, 467–74
5. Auslender, R., Atlas, I., Lissak, A., Bornstein, J., Atad, J. and Abramovici, H. (1996). Follow-up of small, postmenopausal ovarian cysts using vaginal ultrasound and CA-125 antigen. *J. Clin. Ultrasound*, **24**, 175–8
6. Kurjak, A. and Kupesic, S. (1995). Transvaginal color Doppler and pelvic tumor vascularity: lessons learned and future challenges. *Ultrasound Obstet. Gynecol.*, **6**, 1–15
7. Kurjak, A., Predanic, M., Kupesic, S. and Zalud, I. (1994). Adnexal masses malignant ovarian tumors. In Kurjak, A. (ed.) *An Atlas of Transvaginal Color Doppler*, pp. 291–316. (Carnforth, UK: Parthenon Publishing)
8. Barloon, T. J., Brown, B. P., Abu-Yousef, M. M. and Warnock, N. G. (1996). Paraovarian and paratubal cysts: preoperative diagnosis using transabdominal and transvaginal sonography. *J. Clin. Ultrasound*, **24**, 117–22
9. Kupfer, M. C., Schwimer, S. R. and Lebovic, J. (1992). Transvaginal sonographic appearance of endometriomata: spectrum of findings. *J. Ultrasound Med.*, **11**, 129–33
10. Kurjak, A. and Kupesic, S. (1994). Scoring system for prediction of ovarian endometriosis based on transvaginal color and pulsed Doppler sonography. *Fertil. Steril.*, **62**, 81–8
11. Peterson, W. F., Prevost, E. C., Edmunds, F. T. *et al.* (1955). Benign cystic teratomas of the ovary; a clinicostatistical study of 100 cases with a review of the literature. *Am. J. Obstet. Gynecol.*, **70**, 368–82
12. Caruso, P. A., Marsh, M. R., Minicowitz, S. *et al.* (1971). An intense clinicopathologic study of 305 teratomas of the ovary. *Cancer*, **27**, 348
13. Gallion, H., Van Nagell, J. R., Donaldson, E. S. *et al.* (1983). Immature teratoma of the ovary. *Am. J. Obstet. Gynecol.*, **146**, 361–5
14. Woodruff, J. D., Protos, P. and Peterson, W. F. (1968). Ovarian teratoma. *Am. J. Obstet. Gynecol.*, **102**, 702–15
15. Quinn, S. F., Erickson, S. and Black, W. C. (1985). Cystic ovarian teratomas: the sonographic appearance of the dermoid plug. *Radiology*, **155**, 477–8
16. Guttman, P. H. Jr (1977). In search of the elusive benign cystic ovarian teratoma: application of the ultrasound 'tip of the iceberg' sign. *J. Clin. Ultrasound*, **5**, 403–6
17. Owre, A. and Pedersen, J. F. (1991). Characteristic fat–fluid level at ultrasonography of ovarian dermoid cyst. *Acta Radiol.*, **32**, 317–9
18. Di Meglio, A., Di Meglio, G., Esposito, A. *et al.* (1988). Echo patterns of ovarian dermoid tumor. *Eur. J. Gynecol. Oncol.*, **9**, 242–5
19. Malde, H. M., Kedar, R. P., Chadha, D. *et al.* (1992). Dermoid mesh: a sonographic sign of ovarian teratoma. *Am. J. Roentgenol.*, **159**, 1349–50
20. Cohen, L. and Sabbagha, R. (1993). Echo patterns of benign cystic teratomas by transvaginal ultrasound. *Ultrasound Obstet. Gynecol.*, **3**, 120–3
21. Kupesic, S., Kurjak, A., Pasalic, L. *et al.* (1995). The value of transvaginal color Doppler in the assessment of pelvic inflammatory disease. *Ultrasound Med. Biol.*, **21**, 733–8
22. Kurjak, A., Shalan, H., Kupesic, S. *et al.* (1993). Transvaginal color Doppler sonography in the assessment of pelvic tumor vascularity. *Ultrasound Obstet. Gynecol.*, **3**, 137–54

23. Kurjak, A., Predanic, M., Kupesic-Urek, S. *et al.* (1993). Transvaginal color and pulsed Doppler assessment of adnexal tumor vascularity. *Gynecol. Oncol.*, **50**, 3–9

24. Kurjak, A. and Predanic, M. (1992). New scoring system for prediction of ovarian malignancy based on transvaginal color Doppler sonography. *J. Ultrasound Med.*, **11**, 631–8

25. Timor-Tritsch, I. E., Lerner, J. P., Monteagudo, A. *et al.* (1993). Transvaginal ultrasonographic characterization of ovarian masses by means of color flow-directed Doppler measurements and a morphologic scoring system. *Am. J. Obstet. Gynecol.*, **168**, 909–13

26. Lerner, J. P., Timor-Tritsch, I. E., Federman, A. *et al.* (1994). Transvaginal ultrasonographic characterization of ovarian masses with an improved, weighted scoring system. *Am. J. Obstet. Gynecol.*, **170**, 81–5

27. Schulman, H., Conway, C., Zalud, I. *et al.* (1994). Prevalence in a volunteer population of pelvic cancer detected with transvaginal ultrasound and color flow Doppler. *Ultrasound Obstet. Gynecol.*, **4**, 414–20

28. Bourne, T., Campbell, S., Steer, C. *et al.* (1989). Transvaginal color flow imaging: a possible new screening technique for ovarian cancer. *Br. Med. J.*, **299**, 1367–70

29. Brown, D. L., Frates, M. C., Laing, F. C. *et al.* (1994). Ovarian masses: can benign and malignant lesions be differentiated with color and pulsed Doppler US. *Radiology,* **190**, 333–6

30. Fleischer, A. C., Cullinan, J. A., Peery, C. V. and Jones, H. W. (1996). Early detection of ovarian carcinoma with transvaginal color Doppler ultrasonography. *Am. J. Obstet. Gynecol.*, **174**, 101–6

31. Jain, K. A. (1994). Prospective evaluation of adnexal masses with endovaginal gray-scale and duplex and color Doppler US: correlation with pathologic findings. *Radiology,* **191**, 63–7

32. Hata, K., Hata, T., Manabe, A. *et al.* (1992). A critical evaluation of transvaginal Doppler studies, transvaginal sonography, magnetic resonance imaging, and CA 125 in detecting ovarian cancer. *Obstet. Gynecol.*, **80**, 922–6

33. Weiner, Z., Thaler, I., Beck, D. *et al.* (1992). Differentiating malignant from benign ovarian tumors with transvaginal color flow imaging. *Obstet. Gynecol.*, **79**, 159–62

34. Fleischer, A. C., Cullinan, J. A., Kepple, D. M. *et al* (1993). Conventional and color Doppler transvaginal sonography of pelvic masses: a comparison of relative histologic specificities. *J. Ultrasound Med.*, **12**, 705–12

35. Campbell, S., Bourne, T. H., Reynolds, K. *et al.* (1992). Role of color Doppler in an ultrasound-based screening programme. In Sharp, F., Mason, W. P. and Creasman, W. (eds.) *Ovarian Cancer*, Vol. 2, pp. 237–47. (London: Chapman & Hall Medical)

36. Mais, V., Guerriero, S., Ajossa, S. *et al.* (1995). Transvaginal ultrasonography in the diagnosis of cystic teratoma. *Obstet. Gynecol.*, **85**, 48–52

Malignant adnexal masses

5

A. Kurjak, M. Predanic, A. Fleischer and S. Kupesic

Since the introduction of transvaginal color Doppler sonography (TVCD) in the assessment of ovarian vascularity[1,2], attitudes concerning its usefulness in the detection of adnexal malignancies have been equally divided. The majority of the published studies on this subject agree that malignant ovarian tumors, in comparison with benign ones, have characteristic blood flow features. However, overlap in blood flow parameters between malignant and benign ovarian tumors is a main element of the current debate regarding attempts to achieve accurate differentiation of ovarian tumors on the basis of their vascular characteristics. A review of the literature from 1989 to the present[3-35] showed a clear difference between malignant and benign adnexal masses. Those articles revealed high sensitivity and specificity of the newly introduced diagnostic tool and provided a description of malignant adnexal lesions as highly vascular tumors with significantly low vascular resistance to blood flow. Conversely, benign lesions had scant blood supply with high resistance in barely detected tumor vessels. However, over succeeding years, an increasing number of publications have demonstrated a significant overlap in the results and the fact that a large number of benign masses have blood flow features equal to those of malignant lesions and vice versa. The previously built belief that TVCD is valuable and gives strong support in clinical decision making and management has been challenged.

For the purpose of this chapter, we analyzed 33 articles from 27 different institutions in 14 countries worldwide published since 1989[3-35]. Because some institutions have published more than one article on the subject of adnexal vascularity in the last 7 years, or even within 1 year, we chose only one article with the most repre-sentative results from that institution in analyzed years. Table 1 shows the chosen publications on the basis of the aforementioned criteria. The majority of the articles on the assessment of adnexal vascularity and the evaluation of the usefulness of TVCD in the clinical setting were published from 20 departments of obstetrics and gynecology; the other reports were from seven departments of radiology. The largest number of studies (14) were published during 1994. The final conclusion of the articles was evaluated as 'in favor', 'limited use' or 'against' the usefulness of color Doppler in the assessment of adnexal vascularity and the discrimination of malignant vs. benign adnexal lesions. It appears that 51% of the studies were in favor and 19% against the usefulness of TVCD, whereas 30% of the studies evaluated color and pulsed Doppler ultrasound as limited for use in the assessment of adnexal lesions. Again, the largest number of studies that opposed the usefulness of color Doppler were published in 1994.

Table 2 presents the observed results in terms of the screening parameters: sensitivity, specificity, positive predictive value (PPV) and negative predictive value (NPV) from the chosen 33 studies. It is clear that the sensitivity and specificity of the method has significantly decreased since its introduction. A significant reduction of the method's sensitivity and specificity could be explained by several facts. First, TVCD has been accepted by a large number of institutions for trial and evaluation, but different protocols have been used. Second, different ultrasound machines were in use with different setups, as well as different quality of resolution and color/pulsed Doppler sensitivity.

Additionally, the experience of the ultrasonographers probably also played one of the major roles, as did the general attitude and

Table 1 General attitude towards transvaginal color Doppler sonography since 1989

Authors	Year	Department	Number of evaluated tumors	Attitude
Hata et al.[3]	1989	Gynecology	21	in favor
Fleischer et al.[4]	1991	Radiology	43	in favor
Kurjak et al.[5]	1991	Gynecology	680	in favor
Weiner et al.[6]	1992	Gynecology	53	in favor
Kawai et al.[7]	1992	Gynecology	24	in favor
Tekay and Jouppila[8]	1992	Gynecology	72	against
Hata et al.[9]	1992	Gynecology	64	against
Kurjak et al.[10]	1992	Gynecology	83	in favor
Schneider et al.[11]	1993	Gynecology	55	in favor
Hamper et al.[12]	1993	Radiology	31	limited
Timor-Tritsch et al.[13]	1993	Gynecology	115	in favor
Jain[14]	1994	Radiology	50	limited
Weiner et al.[15]	1994	Gynecology	18	in favor
Levine et al.[16]	1994	Radiology	35	against
Brown et al.[17]	1994	Radiology	44	limited
Valentin et al.[18]	1994	Gynecology	149	against
Bromley et al.[19]	1994	Gynecology	33	limited
Carter et al.[20]	1994	Gynecology	30	limited
Prompeler et al.[21]	1994	Gynecology	83	limited
Chou et al.[22]	1994	Gynecology	108	in favor
Wu et al.[23]	1994	Gynecology	410	in favor
Zaneta et al.[24]	1994	Gynecology	76	in favor
Salem et al.[25]	1994	Radiology	102	against
Sengoku et al.[26]	1994	Gynecology	28	in favor
Sawicki et al.[27]	1995	Gynecology	65	in favor
Franchi et al.[28]	1995	Gynecology	129	limited
Maly et al.[29]	1995	Gynecology	102	in favor
Stein et al.[30]	1995	Radiology	169	against
Carter et al.[31]	1995	Gynecology	89	limited
Fleischer et al.[32]	1996	Radiology	126	in favor
Buy et al.[33]	1996	Gynecology	132	limited
Rehn et al.[34]	1996	Gynecology	259	limited
Predanic et al.[35]	1996	Gynecology	106	in favor

belief of the facility in the capability of the new ultrasound modality. For example, from 27 facilities, only one radiology department assessed TVCD as a valuable diagnostic tool, whereas six radiology departments had divided attitudes: three described TVCD as a limited improvement to already used diagnostic tools, and the other three radiology facilities found the method completely inferior to conventional ultrasound (Table 3). On the other hand, departments of obstetrics and gynecology found TVCD very helpful (55%), of limited use (30%) and no use at all (15%). This discrepancy can be explained by the general approach towards the use of color Doppler as an adjunct to conventional ultrasound. While departments of obstetrics and gynecology use this new diagnostic tool as an additional element in the clinical assessment of the patient with adnexal disease, the radiologists assess an adnexal lesion solely as an 'object' extracted from the whole picture of the patient with an adnexal disease. They treat the adnexal lesion as a structure which can be visualized, described and reported with insufficient clinical information and without any further involvement in decision making or management.

To examine our hypothesis, we attempted to correlate the menstrual phase in which patients were examined with the reports published by radiology and gynecology departments, assuming that menstrual phase can alter the blood

Table 2 Screening parameters in the reviewed literature. PPV, positive predictive value; NPV, negative predictive value

Authors	Sensitivity	Specificity	PPV	NPV
Hata et al.[3]	100	100	100	100
Fleischer et al.[4]	100	83	73	100
Kurjak et al.[5]	96	99	98	99
Weiner et al.[6]	94	97	94	94
Kawai et al.[7]	88	100		
Tekay and Jouppila[8]	82	72	35	96
Hata et al.[9]	92	53	59	90
Kurjak et al.[10]	96	95	96	95
Schneider et al.[11]	94	56	47	96
Hamper et al.[12]	66	76	40	90
Timor-Tritsch et al.[13]	94	99	94	99
Jain[14]	70	82		
Weiner et al.[15]	86	100	92	100
Levine et al.[16]	25	89		
Brown et al.[17]	100	79		
Valentin et al.[18]	100	53		
Bromley et al.[19]	66	81		
Carter et al.[20]	57	78	68	69
Prompeler et al.[21]	95	86		
Chou et al.[22]	88	92	85	94
Wu et al.[23]	68	97		
Zaneta et al.[24]	91	85		
Salem et al.[25]	79	77	37	96
Sengoku et al.[26]	82	92	93	79
Sawicki et al.[27]	100	94	95	100
Franchi et al.[28]	76	72	68	93
Maly et al.[29]	100			
Stein et al.[30]	43	56	56	
Carter et al.[31]				
Fleischer et al.[32]	92	86	86	98
Buy et al.[33]	71	67	43	87
Rehn et al.[34]	67	53	22	89
Predanic et al.[35]	86	83	32	98

Table 3 A comparison between the attitudes of departments of radiology and departments of gynecology towards transvaginal color Doppler sonography

Attitude	Radiology		Gynecology		Total	
	n	%	n	%	n	%
In favor	1	14	11	55	12	51
Limited usefulness	3	43	6	30	9	30
Against	3	43	3	15	6	19

flow features of the adnexal masses, creating overlaps in results between benign and malignant lesions (Table 2). However, we found no correlation between the reports of the menstrual phase and the final results. From eight studies published by radiologists, five did not report on the menstrual phase (62%), whereas from 25 articles published by gynecologists, 11 studies reported the menstrual phase (44%), but gynecologists nevertheless evaluated TVCD as a useful new diagnostic tool. Therefore, no significant difference in the method, based on the menstrual cycle, in the assessment of adnexal vascularity was found.

This observation brings us back to the general attitude towards the usefulness of color Doppler. This does not seem to depend on the final results, whether they are good or bad, but on how the new knowledge, even sometimes minimal or insignificant in terms of statistics, can be used and applied in the clinical setting. It seems that gynecologists can use this new diagnostic modality more enthusiastically and with more optimism than radiologists.

Keeping in mind that a major criticism by the opponents of color flow Doppler imaging is that it adds little to the overall management of patients with pelvic masses, we will attempt to discuss and evaluate the capabilities, advantages and benefits, as well as the disadvantages and overestimated results produced by the use of transvaginal color and pulsed Doppler sonography in the assessment of adnexal disease. By the end of the chapter, we hope that our data and experience will support the counter-argument to that of the opponents, and show that color Doppler flow imaging gives the clinician useful additional clinical information in determining those patients in whom early intervention is necessary vs. those in whom expectant management can be safely undertaken.

COLOR DOPPLER AND ADNEXAL MALIGNANT DISEASE

The use of color Doppler sonography is based on the well-established hypothesis that unrestricted growth of tumors is dependent upon angiogenesis[36,37]. The growth of new vessels and development of already existing ones are influenced by specific factors that regulate angiogenic activity[38]. Angiogenesis as a physiological phenomenon can be seen in the endometrium during the process of implantation[39] or in the ovary during folliculogenesis[40]. However, it also occurs as a pathological process during oncogenesis[36]. Most tumors larger than 2–3 mm cannot grow further without the support of vascularization[41]. The development of an adequate vascular network and blood nourishment is crucial to the growth and development as well as the metastasis of a cancer[42]. There is more information about angiogenesis in Chapters 3 and 9. Studies on angiogenesis have shown that the tumor vasculature consists of the vessel recruited from the existing vascular network and vessels that have developed as the angiogenic response of the host vasculature to angiogenesis factors synthesized by cancer cells. Tumor vascularity tends to arise from the venous rather than the arterial host vasculature. Therefore, compared to the normal vessel architecture, blood vessels located at the advancing cancer front lack a muscular coating and consist mostly of an endothelial lining and may contain tumor cells. Because of this characteristic architecture of the tumor blood vessels, tumor vascularization can be analyzed in terms of vessel location, vessel arrangement and pulsed Doppler waveform signal features – shape and resistance to blood flow.

PRESENCE OF BLOOD VESSELS AND VESSEL LOCATION

Macroscopically, the tumor vasculature can be categorized as peripheral or central vascularization[4]. Although this classification is not anatomically correct, it may help in the assessment of the ultrasonically detectable vascular position within tumor tissue. It is believed that peripherally located vessels originate from the pre-existing host vasculature, whereas centrally located vessels develop in response to angiogenic tumor cell activity and/or to necrotic processes. Vessels displayed within septae or papillae represent specific intratumoral branches. The vascular network might be used as an indicator of peripheral blood perfusion of the tumor and its growth, especially in cases of papillary projections. When the vasculature of benign adnexal lesions is correlated with that of malignant lesions, it is found that benign adnexal masses are mostly vascularized pericystically and peripherally, whereas in malignant tumors centrally located vascularization is present most frequently[43]. Although the position of the neovascularization area within tumor tissue is unpredictable, the largest number of blood vessels can be seen in the center of the malignant tumor, peripheral neovascularization being found less often[29] (Figure 1).

Additionally, the presence of color flow in the regular wall or septa does not indicate malignancy, although it can be randomly seen[33].

Color Doppler sonography has the potential to discriminate malignant from benign masses in cases with 'doubtful' morphology. The usefulness of this method was reported specifically for semi-solid or solid–cystic tumors[5,18]. For example, when malignancy is suggested by morphological features, color Doppler may help to demonstrate vascularization in malignant vegetations of ≥ 1 cm[33]. It was also shown that in malignant tumors that had small vegetations without color flow, solid irregular portions with color flow were found, allowing the diagnosis of malignancy. Therefore, an absence of color flow has been considered to suggest a benign lesion[30]. Indeed, color flow has been seen in virtually all malignant adnexal lesions in most series[2,4,5,12,14,23,25,27,44], although occasionally no flow is detected in malignant tumors[4,7,8,14,17,43]. The explanation for this difference may be sought in the diameter of blood vessels which can be depicted with color Doppler sonography. It was found that in benign adnexal lesions the diameter of vessels ranged from 0.01 to 0.03 mm and the number of vessels per field at magnification 10 was between nine and 12. In borderline tumors, the diameter of vessels ranged from 0.01 to 0.1 mm and the number of vessels per field at magnification 10 was between ten and 20, whereas in malignant tumors, the diameter of vessels ranged from 0.01 to 0.1 mm but the number of vessels per field at the same magnification was between 20 and 30[33].

VESSEL ARRANGEMENT

Very few studies tried to evaluate or quantify the amount of vascularity within the tumor. In one of the early series we described the vessel arrangement as a diffuse or isolated vascular pattern. Diffuse vessel arrangement was categorized as more than one color spot displayed, whereas an isolated vessel was described as only one color spot displayed over the tumor tissue[44]. We found that, compared to isolated vessels, diffuse vessels located within the central solid parts of tumors were almost three times higher in malignant tumors (80%) than in benign lesions (33%), suggesting that the area demonstrating a diffuse vessel pattern contains high angiogenic activity (Figure 2). These findings can be related to the previously described study in which the authors found a significantly larger number of blood vessels per field at magnification 10 in malignant tumors than in benign tumors, 20–30 vs. 8–12 blood vessels, respectively[33].

Therefore, we believe that an objective method, such as a computerized method of quantification, is needed to analyze the likelihood of malignancy on the basis of vessel density. Such a system has been described for

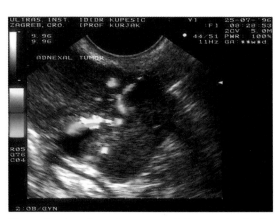

Figure 1 An adnexal mass containing randomly disposed vessels, suggesting high angiogenic activity typical of malignant tumors

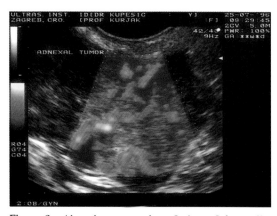

Figure 2 Abundant central perfusion of the malignant tumor is visible with power Doppler technology

predicting the 'vessel density' in nine cases of transplanted murine tumors and has shown excellent correlation with histopathological quantification[45]. The system used seems to provide an accurate depiction of vascularity; time–activity curves showed greater flow in the experimental group injected with exotoxin than in the group injected with saline solution. Vascular density quantification with amplitude color Doppler sonography was shown to be more accurate when an intravascular agent was used.

One of the proposed hypotheses for tumor resistance is poor delivery of chemotherapeutic agents to areas of tumors that are poorly perfused. It is therefore accepted that chemotherapy given simultaneously with an agent that increases blood flow may reach deeper areas of the tumor (which are potentially hypoxic and ischemic) and give better results. The quantification scheme published by Meyerowitz and colleagues[45] may allow the development of a system to assess the malignant potential of the tumor and to monitor the tumor response to chemotherapy on the basis of vascularity of the mass. This technique may be used to assess whether vascular density is a parameter that correlates with the likelihood of the tumor's spread and its metastatic potential. It is expected that three-dimensional imaging conjoined with color Doppler evaluation will depict overall blood flow to the tumor more accurately.

PULSED DOPPLER WAVEFORM

Additional to the localization of blood vessels in the adnexal tumors, it was emphasized that shape of the flow curve is one of the important descriptive data of blood hemodynamics (Figure 3). Appearance of the early diastolic notch or indentation of the early diastolic part of the pulsed Doppler waveform signal slope has been found more often in blood vessels of benign rather than malignant lesions[29,46]. Experimental work with tumors inoculated into rabbit flanks shows that the vessels within areas of active tumor growth have a paucity of muscular tunica media and simulate sinusoids rather than well-formed arterioles. These sinusoid-like vascular spaces have been observed in liver and

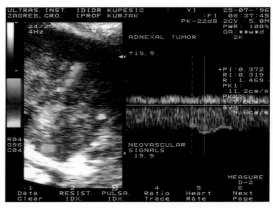

Figure 3 Pulsed Doppler sonogram showing huge diastolic flow and consequently a low impedance value (RI = 0.32). Ovarian malignancy was confirmed by histopathology

ovarian tumors in areas of active tumor growth. The low velocity and impedance waveforms obtained from tumors can be explained on the basis of this type of tumor vessel[47].

In blood vessels with normally developed tunica muscularis, after systole, there is a short period of relaxation of the muscle vessel wall and orthograde flow[47]. This kind of blood flow pattern with an early diastolic notch was demonstrated in the flow curve for ovarian blood vessels during the proliferative phase of the menstrual cycle[3]. Therefore, the lack of a diastolic notch on the waveform is probably related to a lack or relative paucity of smooth muscle in the tunica media, which would account for the initial resistance to flow during the first part of diastole, followed by a relaxation of the muscular wall and forward flow[48].

It must be remembered that a diastolic notch can also be observed at a branch point of vessels. It has also been observed that new vessels found in the wall of a corpus luteum demonstrate the lack of a diastolic notch, perhaps due to the relative lack of a muscular coat in these newly formed vessels[4] (Figure 4). It seems that an early diastolic notch, although a common finding in benign cystic lesions, can also be observed in 7% of malignant multilocular solid tumors[18]. Furthermore, Parsons reported that the vascular wreath within the wall of a corpus lutem was fed by a few larger vessels. Interestingly, the flow in

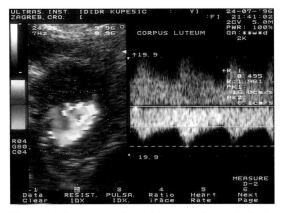

Figure 4 Demonstration of increased vascularity in the corpus luteum (left), with low resistance index (RI = 0.49), representing the typical flow pattern of a corpus luteum (right)

the 'feeding' vessel had higher impedance and velocity than the more distal branches[49].

VASCULAR RESISTANCE TO BLOOD FLOW

It is clear that conflicting attitudes towards Doppler ultrasound in evaluation of vascular characteristics of malignant adnexal masses arise from the largely different results obtained from a number of the studies published in the last several years. It is also important to stress that pulsed Doppler analysis and vascular resistance to blood flow were and still are one of the major features in the assessment of tumor vascular characteristics. Therefore, the earliest and the most recent studies have concentrated on differences of vascular resistance to blood flow between benign and malignant adnexal masses. It has become clear that three groups of investigators can be distinguished.

The first group presented results with high sensitivity and specificity for pulsed Doppler data[4–7,13,22–24,26,27,32,35] with the opinion that this modality significantly improved the accuracy of B-mode ultrasonography, but that the value of this technique in screening procedures should continue to be evaluated.

The second group of investigators was less optimistic in the interpretation of their results[9,11,12,14,17,20,21], stating that Doppler sonography has some potential but currently does not significantly facilitate the decision-making process in routine clinical work.

Finally, a third group of researchers[8,16,19,34] believe that Doppler ultrasound brings nothing new to current diagnostic procedures. They evaluated the technique by itself rather than discussing the possibility that human skill in performing the procedure and poor selection of patients may have been the problem.

It is also interesting to note that the first group of authors began to use the pulsed Doppler technique in its early stage of development when unsophisticated machines were in use but still provided the highest sensitivity and specificity in the evaluation of malignant adnexal masses. It might be considered that uncritical enthusiasm contributed to their optimistic results. Nevertheless, it can be argued that the most powerful tool of this group is their experience in the use of this ultrasound modality, because they continued to publish studies with equally good results[15,32,43,46,48,50–53]. Later studies found less difference in blood flow data with larger overlap between vascular resistance in benign and malignant lesions. However, it is a fact that a difference in vascularity exists and blood vessels in malignant adnexal lesions show lower resistance to blood flow than those in benign adnexal masses. Table 4 gives an overview of pulsed Doppler results in terms of resistance (RI) or pulsatility (PI) indices. We believe that a major problem in observed overlap is due to the variation of RI and PI results within the same tumor. It was suggested in several reports that such a variation exists in adnexal tumors[6–8,18,43,46] and it was further stressed that the operator's responsibility is highly significant in detection and recording of an appropriate blood vessel resistance when no standardization in pulsed Doppler measurement is present. Therefore, a good basic knowledge of Doppler physics is mandatory as well as skillfulness with Doppler instrumentation. Furthermore, the potential pitfalls and the appearance of artifacts must be understood before this technique is applied to patients.

BLOOD FLOW VELOCITIES

Several authors documented the presence of abnormal flow spectra at the periphery of malignant tumors in terms of high blood flow velocities, establishing a hypothesis that such signals resulted from arteriovenous anastomoses[53,54]; this was later confirmed by several groups[55–59]. It was suggested that a cut-off value of 40 cm/s could be used to distinguish blood flow velocities in malignant vs. benign tumors[60]. However, such high blood flow velocities and cut-off values established for breast malignant tumors were not found in adnexal tumors[4,43]. Table 5 reviews the blood flow velocities reported in several publications. It is of value to stress that only one study[21] reported a significant difference between blood flow velocities of benign and malignant lesions. They found blood flow velocity superior to resistance index as a discriminating modality.

SURGICAL STAGE OF MALIGNANT TUMORS

Angiogenesis is a common phenomenon in malignant ovarian neoplasms, but the intensity of neovascularization may depend on individual tumor characteristics[61]. Therefore, an incremental decrease of the impedance indices in adnexal tumors may reflect the increase in angiogenesis intensity as an indication of malignant potential[62]. Animal models showed that

Table 4 Vascular resistance to blood flow, in terms of resistance (RI) or pulsatility (PI) indices, between malignant and benign adnexal lesions

Authors	Index	Malignant adnexal tumors	Benign adnexal tumors
Hata et al.[3]	RI	0.469 ± 0.11	0.96 ± 0.17
Fleischer et al.[4]	PI	0.3–1.5	0.6–4.0
Kawai et al.[7]	PI	0.53 ± 0.65	1.44 ± 0.05
Tekay and Jouppila[8]	PI	0.5 (0.5–0.9)	0.6 (0.5–3.5)
Hata et al.[9]	RI	0.50 ± 0.11	0.69 ± 0.18
Kurjak et al.[10]	RI	0.38 (0.27–0.61)	0.52 (0.46–1.0)
Schneider et al.[11]	RI	0.52 (0.2–1.0)	0.84 (0.24–1.0)
Hamper et al.[12]	RI	0.5 ± 0.17 (0.27–0.67)	0.77 ± 0.33 (0.2–1.0)
Timor-Tritsch et al.[13]	RI	0.39 (0.2–0.53)	0.63 (0.23–0.98)
Levine et al.[16]	RI	0.47 ± 0.11	0.57 ± 0.17
Brown et al.[17]	RI	0.39 ± 0.09 (0.25–0.50)	0.62 ± 0.16 (0.34–0.90)
Valentin et al.[18]	PI	0.9–0.94	0.18–0.96
Carter et al.[20]	RI	0.6 ± 0.1	0.7 ± 0.2
Prompeler et al.[21]	RI	0.40 (0.22–0.66)	0.68 (0.26–1.0)
Chou et al.[22]	RI	0.41 (0.18–0.68)	0.68 (0.36–0.89)
Zaneta et al.[24]	RI	0.46 ± 0.10 (0.27–0.99)	0.72 ± 0.14 (0.43–0.90)
Salem et al.[25]	PI	0.82 ± 0.38 (0.3–1.89)	1.44 ± 0.65 (0.3–3.5)
Sengoku et al.[26]	PI	0.57 ± 0.14	2.42 ± 0.67
Franchi et al.[28]	RI	0.49 (0.28–0.78)	0.72 (0.48–0.98)
Maly et al.[29]	RI	0.5 (0.3–0.6)	0.7 (0.5–1.0)
Stein et al.[30]	RI	0.53 ± 0.16 (0.27–0.83)	0.65 ± 0.18 (0.27–0.98)
Buy et al.[33]	RI	0.54 ± 0.11 (0.28–0.77)	0.59 ± 0.14 (0.34–1.0)
Predanic et al.[35]	RI	0.33 ± 0.03 (0.23–0.45)	0.57 ± 0.02 (0.35–1.0)

Table 5 Blood flow velocities (cm/s) in malignant and benign ovarian tumors

Authors	Malignant adnexal tumors	Benign adnexal tumors
Fleischer et al.[4]	7–61	16–37
Kurjak et al.[43]	14.4–26.2	20.2–27.3
Carter et al.[20]	13.8 ± 10.7	14.4 ± 9.9
Prompeler et al.[21]	47.1 (14.6–105)	17.5 (5.2–61.5)

angiogenesis could be detected by Doppler ultrasound even in a small volume of malignant tumor (25 mg)[63]. This evidence implied that angiogenesis could be detected with current color Doppler ultrasound even when the carcinoma was well confined within the ovarian capsule or exhibited only low malignant potential. Indeed, several series showed that color and pulsed Doppler sonography can depict ovarian carcinoma at stage I[2,64,65] (Figure 5). One series detected two from 18 stage I ovarian carcinomas solely by the presence of an abnormal blood flow pattern in normal-sized ovaries[64], whereas another study found three from 17 stage I cancers on the basis of abnormal blood flow[65]. However, in the latter study, two stage I tumors did not demonstrate flow and both were > 15 cm in size. It could be argued that these undiscovered malignant tumors had a low malignant potential to induce an angiogenic response, or that the blood vessels were so small that they were impossible to depict with current color and pulsed Doppler sensitivity.

The newly developed power or energy modes of color Doppler imaging afford depiction of even smaller vessels but, paradoxically, small intraparenchymal arterioles in benign and normal tissues may show low impedance and a low-velocity blood flow pattern, causing false-positive results. Nevertheless, the tendency towards an incremental decrease in the vascular impedance from benign lesions, borderline malignancy and early malignancy to advanced malignancies was reported[62]. This observation is strongly supported by an *in vivo* study which showed that a similar gradual rise in vascularity with tumor progression in the melanocytic system could be seen[66] with a histopathological approach. This *in vivo* information is in agreement with the notion that an increased vascular supply may facilitate tumorigenesis and aggressive biological behavior in a neoplastic system.

However, as mentioned before, the vascular impedance measured in the parenchymal vessels of an adnexal tumor will not always represent the microangiogenesis itself[67]. Therefore, it is possible that the signal obtained by color and pulsed Doppler demonstrates the main neovascularized channel representing the summation of downstream resistance of the vascular bed in certain tissue block. Additionally, blood flow parameters are not only a result of numerous blood vessels and their wall structure, but also of increased permeability of the analyzed vascular network. Because of increased permeability, stasis of blood flow and short shunts with low impedance can occur, not necessarily being the same in all parts of the tumor[68] (Figure 6).

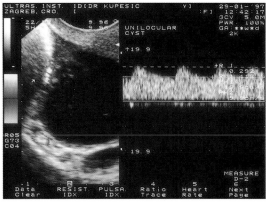

Figure 5 Color flow and pulsed Doppler signals displayed from the dilated vessels in close proximity to the ovarian cyst (left). The low impedance to blood flow (RI = 0.29) which was obtained during the early follicular phase in two subsequent menstrual cycles indicated ovarian malignancy. The small cystic structure proved to be ovarian carcinoma stage Ia

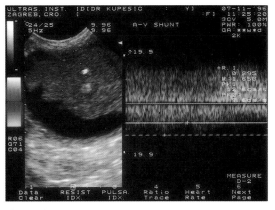

Figure 6 Newly formed vessels produced within the solid part of the complex adnexal tumor, creating the potential for its proliferation and growth. These vessels are deficient in muscular elements, and therefore present diminished resistance to flow (RI = 0.39). Arteriovenous shunts occur at sites of high-pressure gradients and are pathognomonic of malignancy

Increased interstitial pressure is another parameter that may elevate vascular impedance as well as malignant potential.

FALSE-POSITIVE RESULTS

We have shown that, although there is a significant difference in vascular characteristics between benign and malignant adnexal lesions, an overlap in findings can also be expected. This overlap in results can be reduced by adequate knowledge of ultrasound physics and vascular changes through the menstrual cycle, as well as understanding of the morphological characteristics of certain adnexal tumors. Furthermore, the sonographer should be aware that an overlap is characteristic of any biological system. However, even an experienced ultrasonographer using sensitive equipment will not escape the occasional misinterpretation of the ultrasound and Doppler information in equivocal cases. False results can also be caused by increased vascularity in some physiological conditions. An increased blood flow and significantly decreased impedance to blood flow distal to the point of sampling can be seen in a preovulatory follicle and corpus luteum, suggesting that vascular information derived from the premenopausal ovary must always be related to the phase of the cycle.

A ring of angiogenesis around the dominant follicle is most prominent at the moment of the presumed ovulation. The velocity of the perifollicular blood flow tends to increase, while the resistance to blood flow decreases[69]. With the rupture of the follicle and formation of the corpus luteum, angiogenesis continues and further dilatation of the stromal ovarian vessels occurs. The physiological corpus luteum and its variants are frequent false-positive conditions in distinguishing between ovarian malignancy because of abundant and prominent blood flow. Luteal vascularity, described as 'a ring of fire', is probably a consequence of marked dilatation of stromal ovarian blood vessels or 'vascular luteal conversion'[70] due to increased local levels of estradiol prostaglandins, which are known to be potent vasodilators[71,72]. Additional confusion in assessment of luteal blood flow is produced by a

cystic structure with irregular walls of various types and intracystic echoes (Figure 7). Therefore, an irregular cystic structure with echogenic fluid within the cavity, increased blood flow velocity and decreased resistance to blood flow may lead the sonographer to an incorrect interpretation (Figure 8).

Accordingly, physiological ovarian angiogenic activity should be excluded by carrying out the examination during the early proliferative phase of the menstrual cycle. However, this seems not to be completely certain, because some corpus luteum activity and consequently increased ovarian vascularity can be observed in

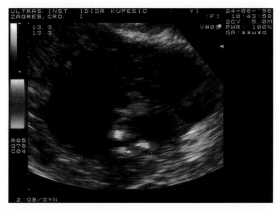

Figure 7 Transvaginal sonogram of a non-specific corpus luteum cyst. Note the greatly dilated vascular channels penetrating the hemorrhagic cavity of the ruptured follicle

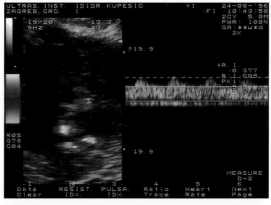

Figure 8 Abundant color flow indicates active corpus luteum. Low resistance index (RI = 0.38) derived from area of angiogenesis may be wrongly interpreted as ovarian malignancy

the first 5 days of the menstrual cycle[72]. Therefore, the corpus luteum and its blood flow should be carefully avoided, as a false-positive diagnosis of ovarian malignancy could be made. The remainder of benign adnexal lesions that may cause false-positive results are tubo-ovarian masses and endometriomas, both entities in which rich vascularity is usually triggered by inflammation[73,74]. In addition, hormonal imbalances in overweight patients can produce blood flow patterns with a low resistance index[75,76].

CONCLUSION

Color and pulsed Doppler sonography visualizes the vascularity of an adnexal mass, providing insight into tumor histology and metabolism. Therefore, blood flow data should be considered to indicate the angiogenic intensity of a tumor, rather than indicating malignancy itself. It seems clear that initial attempts to classify ovarian tumors solely on the basis of their impedance to blood flow have been too simplistic. This problem has been partly solved with the introduction of other vascular parameters such as blood vessel arrangement and location, shape of the pulsed Doppler and appearance of an early diastolic notch, as well as assessment of blood flow velocities.

However, the difference in flow parameters in benign vs. malignant lesions may not always be sufficient to give a firm diagnostic impression. A common criticism of color Doppler is that the operator is never blind to the B-mode image; there is a tendency to search harder for low-impedance blood flow patterns in lesions with a malignant appearance than in simple adnexal cysts. However, when applied by expert operators and in disciplined fashion, it may significantly add to diagnostic information about an adnexal mass and its morphological appearance. If blood flow data are treated as an insight into the tumor's pathology, they give reassurance for those masses with benign appearance while giving confirmation of malignancy in adnexal masses with suspicious morphological features.

References

1. Kurjak, A., Zalud, I., Jurkovic, D., Alfirevic, Z. and Miljan, M. (1989). Transvaginal color Doppler of the assessment of pelvic circulation. *Acta Obstet. Gynecol. Scand.*, **68**, 131–6
2. Bourne, T. H., Campbell, S., Steers, C. V., Whitehead, M. I. and Collins, W. P. (1989). Transvaginal colour flow imaging: a possible new screening technique for ovarian cancer. *Br. Med. J.*, **299**, 1367–70
3. Hata, T., Hata, K., Senoh, D., Makihara, K., Aoki, S., Takamiya, O. and Kitao, M. (1989). Doppler ultrasound assessment of tumor vascularity in gynecologic disorders. *J. Ultrasound Med.*, **8**, 309–14
4. Fleischer, A. C., Rodgers, W. H., Rao, B. J., Keppler, D. M., Worrell, J. A., Williams, L. and Jones, H. W. III. (1991). Assessment of ovarian tumor vascularity with transvaginal color Doppler sonography. *J. Ultrasound Med.*, **10**, 563–8
5. Kurjak, A., Zalud, I. and Alfirevic, Z. (1991). Evaluation of adnexal masses with transvaginal color ultrasound. *J. Ultrasound Med.*, **10**, 295–7
6. Weiner, Z., Thaler, I., Beck, D., Rottem, S., Deutsch, M. and Brandes, J. M. (1992). Differentiating malignant from benign ovarian tumors with transvaginal color flow imaging. *Obstet. Gynecol.*, **79**, 159–62
7. Kawai, M., Kano, T., Kikkawa, F., Maeda, O., Oguchi, H. and Tomoda, Y. (1992). Transvaginal Doppler ultrasound with color flow imaging in the diagnosis of ovarian cancer. *Obstet. Gynecol.*, **79**, 163–7
8. Tekay, A. and Jouppila, P. (1992). Validity of pulsatility and resistance indices in classification of adnexal tumors with transvaginal color Doppler ultrasound. *Ultrasound Obstet. Gynecol.*, **2**, 338–44
9. Hata, H., Hata, T., Manabe, A., Sugimura, K. and Kitao, M. (1992). A critical evaluation of transvaginal Doppler studies, transvaginal sonography, magnetic resonance imaging and CA 125 in detecting ovarian cancer. *Obstet. Gynecol.*, **80**, 922–6
10. Kurjak, A., Schulman, H., Sosic, A., Zalud, I. and Shalan, H. (1992). Transvaginal ultrasound,

color flow, and Doppler waveform of the post-menopausal adnexal mass. *Obstet. Gynecol.*, **80**, 917–21

11. Schneider, V. L., Schneider, A., Reed, K. L. and Hatch, K. D. (1993). Comparison of Doppler with two-dimensional sonography and CA 125 for prediction of malignancy of pelvic masses. *Obstet. Gynecol.*, **81**, 983–8

12. Hamper, U. M., Sheth, S., Abbas, F. M., Rosenshein, B. N., Aronson, D. and Kurman, J. R. (1993). Transvaginal color Doppler sonography of adnexal masses: differences in blood flow impedance in benign and malignant lesions. *Am. J. Roentgenol.*, **160**, 1225–8

13. Timor-Tritsch, I. E., Lerner, J. P., Monteagudo, A. and Santos, R. (1993). Transvaginal ultra-sonographic characterization of masses by means of color flow-directed Doppler measurements and a morphologic scoring system. *Am. J. Obstet. Gynecol.*, **168**, 909–13

14. Jain, K. A. (1994). Prospective evaluation of adnexal masses with endovaginal gray-scale and dupler and color Doppler US: correlation with pathologic findings. *Radiology*, **191**, 63–7

15. Weiner, Z., Beck, D. and Brandes, J. M. (1994). Transvaginal sonography, color flow imaging, computed tomography scanning, and CA 125 as a routine follow-up examination in women with pelvic tumor: detection of recurrent disease. *J. Ultrasound Med.*, **13**, 37–41

16. Levine, D., Feldstein, V. A., Babcook, C. J. and Filly, R. A. (1994). Sonography of ovarian masses: poor sensitivity of resistive index for identifying malignant lesions. *Am. J. Roentgenol.*, **162**, 1355–9

17. Brown, D. L., Frates, M. C., Laing, F. C., DiSalvo, D. N., Doubilet, P. M., Benson, C. B., Waitzkin, E. D. and Muto, M. G. (1994). Ovarian masses: can benign and malignant lesions be differentiated with color and pulsed Doppler US? *Radiology*, **190**, 333–6

18. Valentin, L., Sladkevicius, P. and Marsal, K. (1994). Limited contribution of Doppler velocimetry to the differential diagnosis of extrauterine pelvic tumors. *Obstet. Gynecol.*, **83**, 425–33

19. Bromley, B., Goodman, H. and Benacerraf, B. R. (1994). Comparison between sonographic morphology and Doppler waveform for the diagnosis of ovarian malignancy. *Obstet. Gynecol.*, **83**, 434–7

20. Carter, J., Saltzman, A., Hartenbach, E., Fowler, J., Carson, L. and Twiggs, L. B. (1994). Flow characteristics in benign and malignant gynecologic tumors using transvaginal color flow Doppler. *Obstet. Gynecol.*, **83**, 125–30

21. Prompeler, H. J., Sauerbrei, W. M., Latternann, U. and Pfeiderer, A. (1994). Quantitative flow measurements for classification of ovarian tumors by transvaginal color Doppler sonography in postmenopausal patients. *Ultrasound Obstet. Gynecol.*, **4**, 406–13

22. Chou, C. Y., Chang, C. H., Yao, B. L. and Kuo, H. C. (1994). Color Doppler ultrasonography and serum CA 125 in the differentiation of benign and malignant ovarian tumors. *J. Clin. Ultrasound*, **22**, 491–6

23. Wu, C. C., Lee, C. N., Chen, T. M., Lai, J. I., Hsieh, C. Y. and Hsieh, F. J. (1994). Factors contributing to the accuracy in diagnosing ovarian malignancy by color Doppler ultrasound. *Obstet. Gynecol.*, **84**, 605–8

24. Zaneta, G., Vergani, P. and Lissoni, A. (1994). Color Doppler ultrasound in the preoperative assessment of adnexal masses. *Acta Obstet. Gynecol. Scand.*, **73**, 637–41

25. Salem, S., White, L. M. and Lai, J. (1994). Doppler sonography of adnexal masses: the predictive value of the pulsatility index in benign and malignant disease. *Am. J. Roentgenol.*, **163**, 1147–50

26. Sengoku, K., Satoh, T., Saitoh, S., Abe, M. and Ishikawa, M. (1994). Evaluation of transvaginal color Doppler sonography, transvaginal sonography and CA 125 for prediction of ovarian malignancy. *Int. J. Gynecol. Obstet.*, **46**, 39–43

27. Savicki, E., Spiewankiewicz, B., Cendrowski, K. and Stelmachow, J. (1995). Transvaginal Doppler ultrasound with colour flow imaging in benign and malignant ovarian lesions. *Clin. Exp. Obstet. Gynecol.*, **22**, 137–42

28. Franchi, M., Beretta, P., Ghezzi, F., Zanaboni, F., Goddi, A. and Salvator, S. (1995). Diagnosis of pelvic masses with transabdominal color Doppler, CA 125 and ultrasonography. *Acta Obstet. Gynecol. Scand.*, **75**, 734–9

29. Maly, Z., Riss, P. and Deutinger, J. (1995). Localization of blood vessels and qualitative assessment of blood flow in ovarian tumors. *Obstet. Gynecol.*, **85**, 33–6

30. Stein, S. M., Laifer-Narin, S., Johnson, M. B., Roman, L. D., Muderspach, L. I., Tyszka, J. M. and Ralls, P. W. (1995). Differentiation of benign and malignant adnexal masses: relative value of gray-scale, color Doppler, and spectral Doppler sonography. *Am. J. Roentgenol.*, **164**, 381–6

31. Carter, J. R., Lau, M., Fowler, J. M., Carlson, J. W., Carson, L. F. and Twiggs, L. B. (1995). Blood flow characteristics of ovarian tumors: implications for ovarian cancer screening. *Am. J. Obstet. Gynecol.*, **172**, 901–7

32. Fleischer, A. C., Cullinan, J. A., Peery, C. V., Jones, H. W. III. (1996). Early detection of ovarian carcinoma with transvaginal color Doppler ultrasonography. *Am. J. Obstet. Gynecol.*, **174**, 101–6

33. Buy, J. N., Ghossain, M. A., Hugol, D., Hassen, K., Sciot, C., Truc, J. B., Poitout, P. and Vadrot, D. (1996). Characterization of adnexal masses: combination of color Doppler and conventional sonography compared with spectral Doppler analysis alone and conventional sonography alone. *Am. J. Roentgenol.*, **166**, 385–93

34. Rehn, M., Lohmann, K. and Rempen, A. (1996). Transvaginal ultrasonography of pelvic masses: evaluation of B-mode technique and Doppler ultrasonography. *Am. J. Obstet. Gynecol.*, **175**, 97–104

35. Predanic, M., Vlahos, N., Pennisi, J., Moukhtar, M. and Aleem, F. A. (1996). Color and pulsed Doppler sonography, gray-scale imaging and serum CA 125 in the assessment of adnexal disease. *Obstet. Gynecol.*, **88**, 283–8

36. Folkman, J. (1985). Tumor angiogenesis. *Adv. Cancer Res.*, **48**, 2641–5

37. Folkman, J. and Cotran, R. S. (1976). Relation of vascular proliferation to tumor growth. *Int. Rev. Exp. Pathol.*, **16**, 207–12

38. Folkman, J. and Klaysburn, M. (1987). Angiogenic factors. *Science*, **235**, 442–7

39. Jaffe, R. and Warsof, S. L. (1991). Transvaginal color Doppler imaging in the assessment of uteroplacental blood flow in the normal first-trimester pregnancy. *Am. J. Obstet. Gynecol.*, **164**, 781–5

40. Bourne, T. H., Jurkovic, D., Waterstone, J., Campbell, S. and Collins, W. P. (1991). Intrafollicular blood flow during human ovulation. *Ultrasound Obstet. Gynecol.*, **1**, 215–9

41. Jain, R. K. (1987). Transport of molecules across tumor vasculature. *Cancer Metastasis Rev.*, **6**, 559–61

42. Folkman, J., Watson, K., Ingber, D. and Hanahan, D. (1989). Induction of angiogenesis during the transition from hyperplasia to neoplasia. *Nature (London)*, **339**, 58–61

43. Kurjak, A., Predanic, M., Kupesic-Urek, S. and Jukic, S. (1993). Transvaginal color and pulsed Doppler assessment of adnexal tumor vascularity. *Gynecol. Oncol.*, **50**, 3–9

44. Hata, K., Hata, T., Manage, A. and Kitao, M. (1992). Ovarian tumors of low malignant potential: transvaginal Doppler ultrasound features. *Gynecol. Oncol.*, **45**, 259–64

45. Meyerowitz, C. B., Fleischer, A. C., Pickens, D. R., Thurman, G. B., Borowsky, A. D., Thirsk, G. and Hellerqvist, C. G. (1996). Quantification of tumor vascularity and flow with amplitude color Doppler sonography in an experimental model: preliminary results. *J. Ultrasound Med.*, **15**, 827–33

46. Fleischer, A. C., Rodgers, W. H., Kepple, D. M., Williams, L. L., Jones, H. W. III (1993). Color

Doppler sonography of ovarian masses: a multiparameter analysis. *J. Ultrasound Med.*, **12**, 41–8

47. Shubik, P. (1982). Vascularization of tumors: a review. *J. Cancer Res. Clin. Oncol.*, **103**, 211–19

48. Fleischer, A. C., Cullinan, J. A., Jones, H. W. III, Peery, C. V. and Bluth, R. F. (1995). Serial assessment of adnexal masses with transvaginal color Doppler sonography. *Ultrasound Med. Biol.*, **21**, 435–43

49. Parsons, A. K. (1994). Ultrasound of the human corpus luteum. *Ultrasound Q.*, **12**, 127–66

50. Kurjak, A. and Predanic, M. (1992). New scoring system for prediction of ovarian malignancy based on transvaginal color Doppler sonography. *J. Ultrasound Med.*, **11**, 631–8

51. Hata, K., Makihara, K., Hata, T., Takahashi, K. and Kitao, M. (1991). Transvaginal color Doppler imaging for hemodynamic assessment of reproductive tract tumors. *Int. J. Gynecol. Obstet.*, **36**, 301–8

52. Bourne, T. H., Campbell, S., Reynolds, K. M., Whitehead, M. I., Hampson, J., Royston, P., Crayford, T. J. B. and Collins, W. P. (1993). Screening for early familial ovarian cancer with transvaginal ultrasonography and color flow imaging. *Br. Med. J.*, **306**, 1025–9

53. Wells, P. N. T., Halliwell, M., Skidmore, R., Webb, A. J. and Woodcock, J. P. (1977). Doppler studies of the breast. *Ultrasound Med. Biol.*, **15**, 231–5

54. Burns, P. N., Halliwell, M., Webb, A. J. and Wells, P. N. T. (1982). Ultrasonics Doppler studies of the breast. *Ultrasound Med. Biol.*, 127–43

55. Shimamoto, K., Sakuma, S., Ishigaki, T. and Makino, N. (1987). Intratumoral blood flow: evaluation with color Doppler echography. *Radiology*, **165**, 683–5

56. Jellins, J., Kossoff, G., Boyd, J. and Reeve, T. S. (1983). The complementary role of Doppler to the B-mode examination of the breast. *J. Ultrasound Med.*, **10**, 29–35

57. Maniasan, M. and Bamber, J. C. A. (1983). A preliminary assessment of an ultrasonic Doppler method for the study of blood flow in human breast cancer. *Ultrasound Med. Biol.*, **8**, 257–61

58. Taylor, K. J. W. and Morse, S. S. (1988). Doppler detects vascularity of some malignant tumors. *Diagn. Imaging*, **10**, 132–6

59. Taylor, K. J. W., Ramos, I., Carter, D., Morse, S. S., Snower, D. and Fortune, K. (1991). Correlation of Doppler US tumor signals with neovascular morphologic features. *Radiology*, **166**, 57–62

60. Dock, W., Grabanwoger, F., Metz, V., Elbenberger, K. and Farres, M. (1991). Tumor vascularization: assessment with duplex sonography. *Radiology*, **181**, 241–4

61. Bourne, T. H. (1994). Should clinical decisions be made about ovarian masses using transvaginal color Doppler? *Ultrasound Obstet. Gynecol.*, **4**, 257–60

62. Wu, C. C., Lee, C. N., Chen, T. M., Shyu, M. K., Hsieh, C. Y., Chen, H. Y. and Hsieh, F. J. (1994). Incremental angiogenesis assessed by color Doppler ultrasound in the tumorigenesis of ovarian neoplasms. *Cancer,* **73**, 1251–6

63. Ramos, I., Fernandez, L. A., Morse, S. S., Fortune, K. L. and Taylor, K. J. W. (1988). Detection of neovascular signal in a 3-day Walker 256 rat carcinosarcoma by CW Doppler ultrasound. *Ultrasound Med. Biol.*, **14**, 123–6

64. Kurjak, A., Shalan, H., Matijevic, R., Predanic, M. and Kupesic-Urek, S. (1993). Stage I ovarian cancer by transvaginal color Doppler sonography: a report of 18 cases. *Ultrasound Obstet. Gynecol.*, **3**, 195–8

65. Fleischer, A. C., Cullinan, J. A., Peery, C. V. and Jones, J. W. III (1996). Early detection of ovarian carcinoma with transvaginal color Doppler ultrasound. *Am. J. Obstet. Gynecol.*, **174**, 101–6

66. Barnhill, R. L., Fandrey, K., Levy, M. A., Mihm, M. C. Jr and Human, B. (1992). Angiogenesis and tumor progression of melanoma: quantification of vascularity in melanocytic nevi and cutaneous malignant melanoma. *Lab. Invest.,* **67**, 57–62

67. Srivastava, A., Laidler, P., Davies, R. P., Horgan, K. and Hughes, L. E. (1988). The prognostic significance of tumor vascularity in intermediate thickness (0.76–4.0 mm thick) melanoma: a quantitative histologic study. *Am. J. Pathol.,* **133**, 419–23

68. Blood, C. H. and Zetter, B. R. (1990). Tumor interactions with the vasculature: angiogenesis and tumor metastasis. *Biochem. Biophys. Acta,* **1032**, 89–118

69. Kurjak, A., Kupesic, S., Schulman, H. and Zalud, I. (1991). Transvaginal color flow Doppler in the assessment of ovarian and uterine blood flow in infertile women. *Fertil. Steril.,* **56**, 870–3

70. Merce, L. T., Garces, D., Barco, M. J. and de la Fuente, F. (1992). Intraovarian Doppler velocimetry in ovulatory, dysovulatory and anovulatory cycles. *Ultrasound Obstet. Gynecol.,* **2**, 197–202

71. Alila, H. W., Corrandino, R. A. and Hansel, W. (1988). A comparison of the effects of cyclooxygenase prostanoids on progesterone production by small and large bovine luteal cells. *Prostaglandins,* **36**, 259–70

72. Raud, J. (1990). Vasodilatation and inhibition of mediator release represent two distinct mechanisms of prostaglandin modulation of acute mast cell-dependent inflammation. *Br. J. Pharmacol.,* **99**, 449–54

73. Sladkevicius, P., Valentin, L., and Marsal, K. (1994). Blood flow velocity in the uterine and ovarian arteries during menstruation. *Ultrasound Obstet. Gynecol.,* **4**, 421–7

74. Kupesic, S., Kurjak, A., Pasalic, L. and Benic, S. (1995). Transvaginal color Doppler in the assessment of pelvic inflammatory disease. *J. Ultrasound Med. Biol.,* **6**, 733–8

75. Kurjak, A. and Kupesic, S. (1994). Scoring system for prediction of ovarian endometriosis based on transvaginal color and pulsed Doppler sonography. *Fertil. Steril.,* **62**, 81–8

76. Aleem, F. and Predanic, M. (1996). Transvaginal color Doppler determination of the ovarian and uterine blood flow characteristics in polycystic ovarian disease. *Fertil. Steril.,* **65**, 510–6

Color Doppler sonography in the early detection of ovarian cancer

6

A. C. Fleischer, D. L. Tait and J. E. Johnson

INTRODUCTION

Color Doppler sonography (CDS) has been shown to be a clinically useful adjunct to transvaginal sonography (TVS) for the evaluation of patients with pelvic masses[1–4]. CDS can improve the detection of malignancy by showing low-impedance, high-velocity flow in morphologically abnormal areas. However, false-positive and false-negative diagnoses can occur with CDS. Occasionally, the CDS features may suggest malignancy in morphologically non-suspicious masses. This stresses the importance of the integration of clinical and laboratory information with the CDS findings. CDS is dependent on the operator and equipment, as well as being relatively expensive. These advantages and limitations must be considered when discussing the optimal integration of CDS in screening and/or early detection programs for ovarian cancer[5,6].

This chapter presents data concerning optimization of screening and/or early detection schemes involving CDS. Identification of women at greatest risk for ovarian cancer by clinical history, CA 125 and breast/ovarian cancer genetic analysis (BRCA 1 and 2) is discussed.

FUNDAMENTAL CONCEPTS OF SCREENING AND EARLY DETECTION

There are fundamental concepts that differentiate effective screening tests from those performed as diagnostic studies. Screening implies study of an unselected population for a certain disease, whereas diagnostic studies are performed on selected subjects because of clinical suspicion or the identification of certain risk factors. In order for a screening test to be considered effective, it must detect a disease in which medical treatment can positively affect outcome, have a high degree of sensitivity and specificity, be cost- and effort-effective and be non-invasive[7].

Other factors that influence the effectiveness of screening are intrinsic to the disease. There are a variety of doubling times for various histological types of ovarian carcinoma, making assessment of 'length' and 'time' biases difficult. 'Length time' bias involves differences in the screening outcomes related to the aggressiveness of tumor growth, since some tumors can remain clinically silent for a long time, but others grow quickly. 'Lead time' bias arises if the time of diagnosis of a condition influences outcome. These are both important parameters in consideration of the efficacy of screening for ovarian cancer.

The low annual incidence of ovarian cancer (33 per 100 000 in the USA at age 55) in the general population is the ultimate limitation to screening for ovarian cancer[8]. Other factors that limit the effectiveness of screening include cost and detection of false positives. However, selective evaluation by TVS and CDS of women who are identified to be at high risk has been shown to allow early detection[1,4].

RISK FACTORS AND LABORATORY TESTS

Because the incidence of ovarian cancer is relatively low, screening of the general population is probably not effective[9]. The average age at diagnosis is 57 years, and this also influences the efficacy of screening the entire female

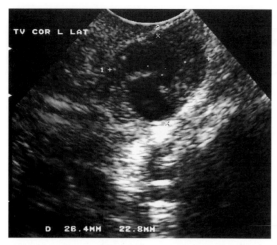

Figure 1 Stage I ovarian cancer: transvaginal sonography (TVS), showing minor irregularity of wall in cystic area within a normal-sized ovary. The morphological findings of ovarian carcinoma can be subtle, such as in this case. However, serial TVS over several months showed a persistent abnormality

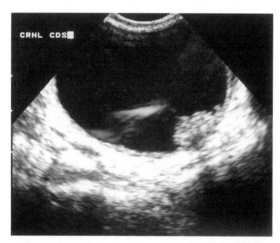

Figure 2 Stage I ovarian cancer: transvaginal sonographic findings. This elderly patient had a cystic mass with a broad-based papillary excrescence. This finding is highly suggestive of an ovarian cancer

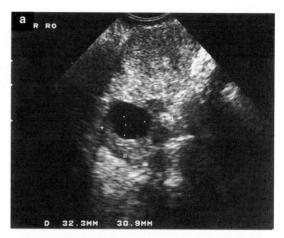

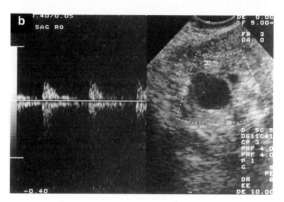

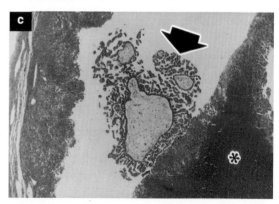

Figure 3 Stage I ovarian cancer. (a) Transvaginal sonography, showing a smooth-walled cystic area within a normal-sized ovary. The patient had a mildly elevated CA 125 level. (b) Transvaginal color Doppler sonography, showing high-impedance flow within the ovary. (c) Low-power (× 4 original magnification) photomicrograph showing microscopic focus of approximately 2 mm of tumor (arrow) adjacent to hemorrhagic area (asterisk)

population. However, close evaluation of women who are identified to be 'at risk' will improve the efficacy of screening schemes.

The lifetime risk for developing ovarian cancer is 1 in 70 (1.4%) for the general population. Nulliparity, perineal talc exposure, infertility, high-fat diet and previous breast cancer infer a 2.0% lifetime risk. Family history of ovarian

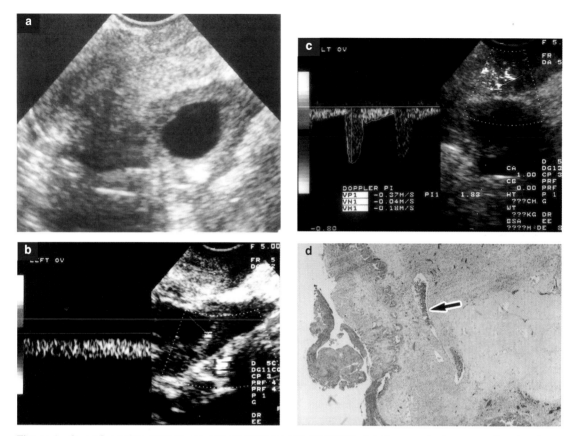

Figure 4 Stage I ovarian cancer: color Doppler sonography (CDS). (a) Transvaginal sonography, showing a thick-walled cyst within a slightly enlarged ovary. (b) Transvaginal CDS, showing low-impedance flow within the wall. (c) Clusters of vessels surrounding the mass. (d) Low-power photomicrograph, showing abnormal 'sinusoidal' tumor vessels (arrow)

cancer increases the risk in one second-degree relative to 2.9%, one first-degree relative to 4.5% and two first-degree relatives to 39%[10].

Studies that utilized TVS and CDS in a selected population have demonstrated efficacy. For example, one study of 1600 women with a family history of ovarian cancer detected six ovarian cancers, five of which were of stage I[3]. Other studies that used CA 125 as the initial screening parameter detected ovarian cancer, but more frequently it was of a later stage[11].

The vast majority (over 90%) of ovarian cancer occurs in women without a family history or known predisposing factor. The ovarian cancer syndromes represent less than 1–3% of all ovarian cancer. They can be subdivided into ovarian site-specific, breast–ovarian and multiple site (Lynch type II – ovarian, proximal colon,

endometrial cancers). These women tend to have ovarian cancer with an earlier age of onset (median 47 years with 20% occurring before 40 years) than the ovarian cancer that occurs in the general population (median 57 years).

The most recent development in genetic testing to identify women at risk for developing breast and ovarian cancer is analysis of the BRCA gene locus on the long arm of chromosome 17. The presence of this gene mutation confers a 30% risk of ovarian cancer by the age of 60 years[12]. Loss of heterogeneity in the BRCA gene has been identified in up to 70% of sporadically occurring ovarian cancers. This gene mutation has been shown to be present in a group of Israeli women with ovarian cancer[13].

It has been estimated that 40–60% of ovarian cancers are associated with malfunction of p53,

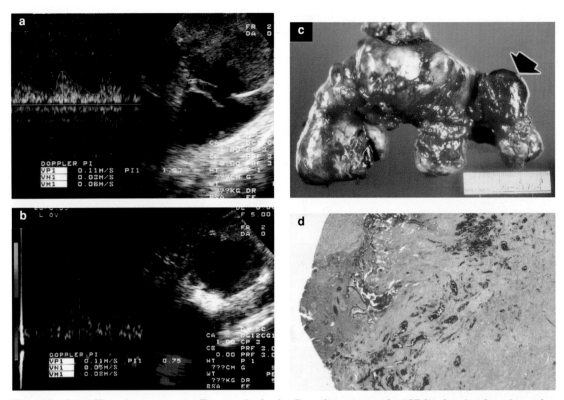

Figure 5 Stage II ovarian cancer. (a) Transvaginal color Doppler sonography (CDS), showing 3 cm irregular solid mass adjacent to distended left tube. High-impedance flow is seen within a vessel coursing in the tube wall. (b) Transvaginal CDS through ovarian mass, showing low-impedance flow. Stage II ovarian cancer. (c) Excised specimen, showing mass (arrow) and adjacent hydrosalpinx. (d) Photomicrograph, showing abnormal vessels within the tumor

a gene locus responsible for tumor growth inhibition[14]. Abnormalities in p53 result in malfunction of tumor inhibition, leading to the development of tumors.

A blood test for the antigen CA 125 can identify malignancies but has relatively limited sensitivity and specificity. Only 50% of stage I cancers were positive in a large series and elevated levels can be seen in a variety of disorders, especially in the premenopausal age group. It is an accurate means to detect recurrent disease, however[15]. New tumor markers such as urinary gonadotropin product (UGP) are being developed and studied[16].

COLOR DOPPLER SONOGRAPHY

It is with these limitations in mind that the use of CDS in screening must be considered.

Clearly, the efficacy of CDS as a means to improve the efficiency of screening is intertwined with efforts at better identification of women at risk.

In one study that examined women with a history of breast cancer, CDS improved sensitivity from 25 to 65% for the detection of ovarian cancer when compared to TVS[17]. The use of CDS improved the odds ratio of finding an ovarian cancer from 1 : 9 to 2 : 5 in women with a familial history of ovarian cancer[3].

In two studies that used TVS and CDS as a means to detect ovarian cancer in the general population, a detection rate of 2 per 1000 was reported[2,18]. When combined with early detection of endometrial cancer, the detection rate was similar to that of mammography for breast cancer (6 per 1000). When TVS was offered to a general population, one gynecologist found

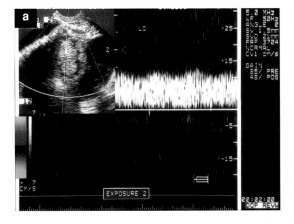

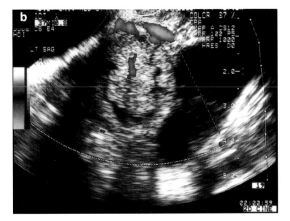

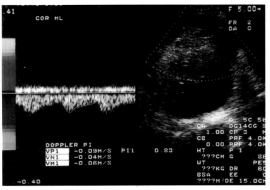

Figure 7 Transvaginal color Doppler sonography, showing low impedance flow within irregular solid area, diagnostic of ovarian cancer. This patient's mass was found prior to a chorionic villus sampling procedure at 9 weeks

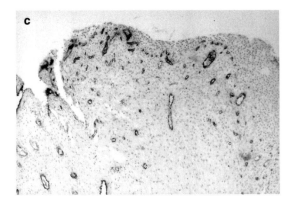

Figure 6 Papillary ovarian cancer within a follicle-containing ovary in a patient undergoing ovulation induction. (a) Transvaginal color Doppler sonography (CDS), showing low-impedance flow within papillary excrescence. There were also two mature follicles within this ovary. (b) Amplitude transvaginal CDS, showing a vessel within the papillary excrescence. (c) Low-power photomicrograph with vessel staining shows highly vascular area within the tumor

one case of ovarian cancer and one case of endometrial cancer in 478 women examined[19]. He also found nine benign ovarian masses and three benign endometrial disorders.

Fortunately, the high degree of vascularity of most early stage tumors improves their detection with CDS, even though the morphological findings may be subtle[1] (Figures 1–6). The extent of vascularity may vary according to the stage of tumor growth (Figures 7 and 8). Even with this factor, a number of investigators have reported detection of early stage tumors with CDS[1,3,4]. Some of these tumors were in only slightly enlarged ovaries.

SUMMARY

The efficacy of screening for ovarian cancer with sonography is inherently limited, owing to the low prevalence of the disease[20]. However, the sonographic evaluation of women who are identified to have increased risk is efficacious and can result in early detection. This requires proper integration of CDS as an adjunct to TVS.

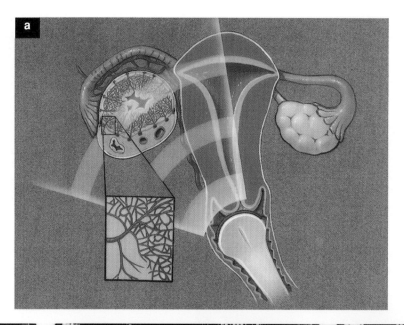

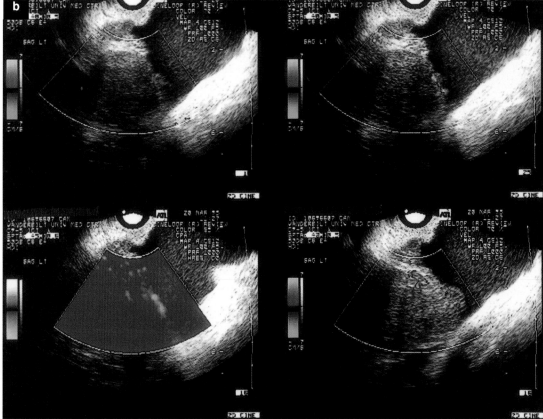

Figure 8 Tumor vascularity. (a) Drawing depicting tumor vascularity in an ovarian tumor (drawing by Paul Gross, MS). (b) Composite transvaginal color Doppler sonography (CDS), showing frequency and amplitude CDS findings in ovarian cancer. (Top left, top right, bottom right) frequency CDS of solid pelvic mass; (bottom left) amplitude CDS showing clustered vessels within the ovarian cancer

References

1. Kurjak, A., Shalan, H., Matijevic, R., Predanic, M. and Kupesic-Urek, S. (1993). Stage I ovarian cancer by transvaginal color Doppler sonography: a report of 18 cases. *Ultrasound Obstet. Gynecol.*, **3**, 195–8

2. Kurjak, A., Shalan, H., Kupesic, S., Kosuta, D., Sosic, A., Benic, S., Ilijas, M., Jukic, S. and Predanic, M. (1994). An attempt to screen asymptomatic women for ovarian and endometrial cancer with transvaginal color and pulsed Doppler sonography. *J. Ultrasound Med.*, **13**, 295–301

3. Bourne, T. H., Campbell, S., Reynolds, K. M., Whitehead, M. I., Hampson, J., Royston, P., Crayford, T. J. B. and Collins, W. P. (1993). Screening for early familial ovarian cancer with transvaginal ultrasonography and colour blood flow imaging. *Br. Med. J.*, **306**, 1025–9

4. Fleischer, A. C., Cullivan, J., Peery, C. and Jones, H. (1996). Early detection of ovarian carcinoma with transvaginal color Doppler ultrasonography. *Am. J. Obstet. Gynecol.*, **174**, 101–6

5. Karlan, B. Y., Raffel, L. J., Crvenkovic, G., Smrt, C., Chen, M. D., Lopez, E., Walla, C. A., Garber, C., Cane, P., Sarti, D. A., Rotter, J. I. and Platt, L. D. (1993). A multidisciplinary approach to the early detection of ovarian carcinoma: rationale, protocol design, and early results. *Am. J. Obstet. Gynecol.*, **169**, 494–501

6. Cohen, C. J. and Jennings, T. S. (1994). Screening for ovarian cancer: the role of noninvasive imaging techniques. *Am. J. Obstet. Gynecol.*, **4**, 1088–94

7. Black, W. C. and Welch, H. G. (1997). Screening for disease. *Am. J. Roentgenol.*, **168**, 3–11

8. Schapira, M. M., Matchar, D. B. and Young, M. J. (1993). The effectiveness of ovarian cancer screening. *Ann. Intern. Med.*, **118**, 838–43

9. van Nagell, J. R., DePriest, P. D., Gallion, H. H. and Pavlik, E. J. (1993). Ovarian cancer screening. *Cancer*, **71**, 1523–8

10. Piver, M. S. and Hempling, R. E. (1993). Etiology and screening of ovarian cancer. *Telinde's Operative Gynecol. Updates*, **1**, 1–13

11. Jacobs, I., Davies, A. P., Bridges, J., Stabile, I., Fay, T., Lower, A., Grudzinskas, J. G. and Oram, D. (1993). Prevalence screening for ovarian cancer in postmenopausal women by CA 125 measurement and ultrasonography. *Br. Med. J.*, **306**, 1030–4

12. Easton, D. F., Ford, D., Bishop, D. T. and the Breast Cancer Linkage Consortium (1995). Breast and ovarian cancer incidence in BRCAI-mutation carriers. *Am. J. Hum. Genet.*, **56**, 265–71

13. Modan, B., Gak, E., Sade-Bruchim, R. B., Hirsh-Yechezkel, G., Theodor, L., Lubin, F., Ben-Baruch, G., Beller, U., Fishman, A., Dgani, R., Menczer, J., Papa, M. and Friedman, E. (1996). High frequency of BRCA1 185delAG mutation in ovarian cancer in Israel. *J. Am. Med. Assoc.*, **276**, 1823–5

14. Takahashi, H., Behbakht, K., McGovern, P.E., Chiu, H., Couch, F. J., Weber, B. L., Friedman, L. S., King, M. C., Furusato, M., LiVolsi, V. A., Menzin, A. W., Liu, P. C., Benjamin, I., Morgan, M. A., King, S. A., Rebane, B. A., Cardonick, A., Mikuta, J. J., Rubin, S. C. and Boyd, J. (1995). Mutation analysis of the BRCA1 gene in ovarian cancers. *Cancer Res.*, **55**, 2998–3002

15. Zurawski, V., Orjaseter, H., Anderson, A. and Jellum, E. (1988). Elevated serum CA-125 levels prior to diagnosis of ovarian neoplasia: relevance for early detection of ovarian cancer. *Int. Cancer*, **42**, 677–80

16. Cane, P., Azen, C., Lopez, E., Platt, L. D. and Karlan, B. Y. (1994). Tumor marker trends in asymptomatic women at risk for ovarian cancer: relevance for ovarian cancer screening. *Gynecol. Oncol.*, 240–5

17. Weiner, Z., Beck, D., Shteiner, M. *et al.* (1993). Screening for ovarian cancer in women with breast cancer with transvaginal sonography and color flow imaging. *J. Ultrasound Med.*, **12**, 387

18. Schulman, H., Conway, C., Zalud, I., Farmakides, G., Haley, J. and Cassata, M. (1994). Prevalence in a volunteer population of pelvic cancer detected with transvaginal ultrasound and color flow Doppler. *Ultrasound Obstet. Gynecol.*, **4**, 414–20

19. Holbert, T. R. (1994). Screening transvaginal ultrasonography of postmenopausal women in a private office setting. *Am. J. Obstet. Gynecol.*, **170**, 1699–704

20. Taylor, K. J. W. and Schwartz, P. E. (1994). Screening for early ovarian cancer. *Radiology*, **192**, 1–10

Color Doppler sonography in pelvic pain

7

A. C. Fleischer

INTRODUCTION

One of the most common problems that the gynecologist deals with is patients with a presenting complaint of pelvic pain. Transvaginal sonography (TVS) alone and with color Doppler sonography (CDS) is an effective means for detecting the location and source of pelvic pain.

There are many causes of pelvic pain, some of which can be detected with imaging techniques, and others which remain uncertain even after laproscopy. One of the most common causes of pelvic pain is associated with hemorrhage into functional ovarian cysts. In one study, only 63% of women undergoing laparoscopy for pelvic pain had abnormal findings[1]. Conversely, 18% of women with pain and abnormal pelvic examinations had no abnormalities at laparoscopy. There is not always a correlation between the presence of pelvic pain and abnormality of the pelvic organs. In this correlative study, ovarian abnormalities accounted for approximately 10% in the series of women with pelvic pain who underwent laparoscopy, 27% had pelvic adhesions, 22% had pelvic inflammatory disease and 3% had unsuspected endometrioma[1].

Those disorders which can be associated with pelvic pain and which will be emphasized in this chapter include:

(1) Adnexal torsion;

(2) Endometriosis/adenomyosis;

(3) Ovarian remnant syndrome;

(4) Ureteral calculi;

(5) Appendicitis and other bowel-related disorders such as ischemic bowel disease; and

(6) Pelvic congestion syndrome.

Other disorders that may be associated with pelvic pain, such as ectopic pregnancy and endometriosis, are covered in other chapters.

ADNEXAL TORSION

Color Doppler sonography has an important role in the evaluation of women presenting with lower abdominal and pelvic pain. In particular, the possibility of adnexal torsion can be assessed by this modality. However, confident and early diagnosis of this entity relies on optimization of scanning techniques such as gray-scale/color write priority settings. If the color/gray-scale priority is not optimized, the absence of flow may be overread. It is always important to assess the opposite ovary for flow, since torsion is usually unilateral and flow is usually detectable in the unaffected ovary.

The importance of recognition of certain flow patterns will be emphasized as they relate to the viability of the ovary once it has undergone torsion.

Clinical features

There are a variety of disorders that result in lower abdominal and pelvic pain. Transvaginal and transabdominal sonography have a pivotal role in distinguishing adnexal causes from non-gynecological causes such as appendicitis or distal ureteral obstruction due to renal calculus[2]. Patients with adnexal torsion may present several times to the emergency department for urgent evaluation[3]. Their symptoms may be attributed to appendicitis, urinary tract infection, inflammatory bowel disease, endometriosis or

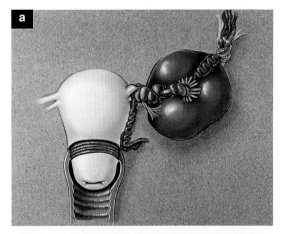

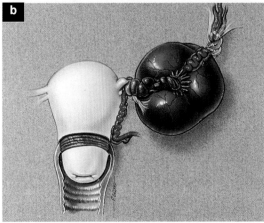

Figure 1 Diagrams showing adnexal (ovarian) torsion in the early (a) and late (b) phase. In the acute phase (first hours) there is engorgement of the ovary and tube, followed by gangrenous changes later. The challenge of imaging specialists is the early and confident diagnosis of adnexal torsion

functional ovulatory pain. It is not uncommon for patients who have the final diagnosis of adnexal torsion to be treated mistakenly for urinary tract infection or other disorders. The pain associated with adnexal torsion is usually intense and localized to either adnexal region. It may be intermittent; this can be attributed to intermittent episodes of incomplete torsion. Expeditious and confident identification of adnexal torsion by CDS may result in salvage of the ovaries and Fallopian tubes (Figure 1).

The pathophysiology torsion varies according to its cause. In some cases, there is massive edema of the ovary probably related to vasodi-

latation with leakage of blood into the ovarian interstitium combined with hindered venous outflow[4]. In others, thrombus within the ovarian vein may contribute to venous engorgement of the ovary, further precipitating torsion. We have documented the presence of thrombi within the smaller intraovarian veins in some cases of torsion. In other cases, torsion is associated with a mass or hemorrhage within the ovary[3]. Some attribute torsion to relatively lax ligamentous support of the ovary, particularly in children[5]. Tubal torsion should be suspected in women who have undergone tubal ligation. The ligated tubal segment may become filled with fluid and be predisposed to torsion. Ovulation stimulation may be associated with enlarged ovaries that contain numerous follicles. These ovaries tend to undergo torsion and quick recognition of this may lead to conservative surgery[6]. Adnexal torsion may also be encountered in pregnant patients and possibly be related to corpus luteum cysts that may persist during pregnancy. Therefore, it is emphasized that adnexal torsion is typically associated with:

(1) Massive edema and/or hemorrhage within the ovary; or

(2) Multiple follicles or corpora lutea associated with ovulation induction; or

(3) Adnexal masses such as ovarian or paraovarian tumors.

Accordingly, torsion is typically seen in either younger patients, in whom it is related to hemorrhage or conditions that increase the 'weight' of the ovary, or older women, in whom it is related to the presence of ovarian or adnexal masses. A third group of patients in whom torsion is seen is women undergoing ovulation induction. Usually, adnexal torsion involves both the tube and ovary.

Sonographic findings

Before discussing the CDS findings in ovarian torsion, one should be aware of the spectrum of CDS findings in normal ovaries. The arterial flow to and within the ovary is dependent on the presence of maturing follicles and corpora

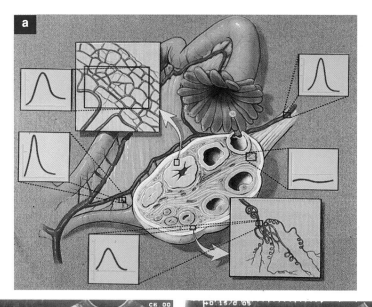

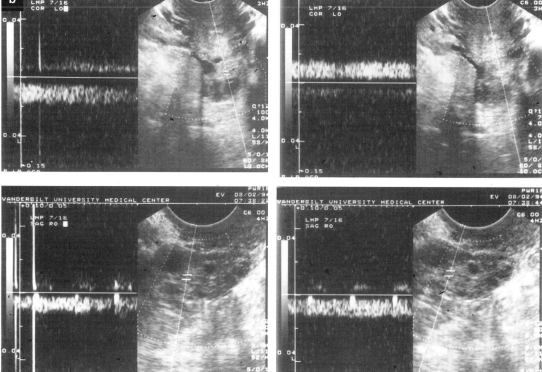

Figure 2 Normal adnexal blood flow. (a) Diagram of arterial flow to the ovary. The ovary is supplied by the main ovarian artery, which branches from the aorta and the adnexal branch of the uterine artery. There are arterial anastomoses with the tubal blood supply as well. Intraovarian arterial flow depends on the proximity to a developing follicle or corpus luteum. Near a corpus luteum, the flow has low resistance and high diastolic flow, whereas in areas away from developing follicles, the intraovarian arterioles are spiral and have high resistance. Venous flow roughly parallels arterial flow. (b) Composite transvaginal color Doppler sonograms, showing intraovarian arterial and venous flow to both normal-sized ovaries, thus negating the possibility of torsion. *Continued on p. 72*

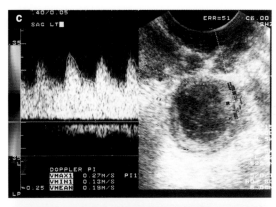

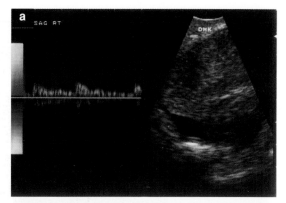

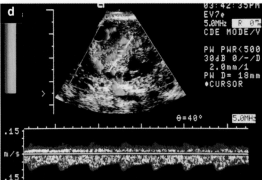

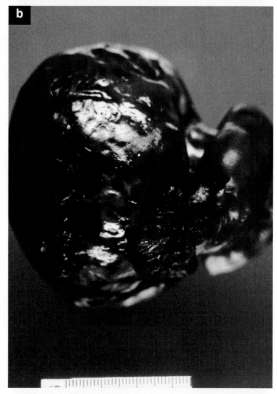

Figure 2 *continued* (c) Low-impedence intraovarian blood flow within the wall of a hemorrhagic corpus luteum. (d) Amplitude color Doppler sonography, showing normal low-impedance flow in the wall of a corpus luteum

lutea. Doppler signals arising from the larger feeding vessels (adnexal branch of uterine and main ovarian artery) should be apparent throughout the cycle and in most postmenopausal women. Intraovarian arteries and arterioles can be seen around the corpus luteum owing to the extensive vascularity of their walls. Venous signals are also seen within the ovary in most patients.

The ovarian blood supply may vary in its predominant flow from either ovarian or uterine circulations. From the larger feeding vessels usually five or six branches or two large branches with multiple twigs pentrate the capsule to supply the ovarian parenchyma (Figure 2). The intraovarian branches are coiled in areas devoid of significant follicular development but are circumferential in areas of maturing follicles. A vascular 'wreath' is seen around functioning corpora lutea.

Figure 3 Enlarged ovary in 18-year-old presenting with 3-day history of acute pelvic pain. A similar episode was experienced 1 and 2 months prior to this admission. (a) Triplex transvaginal color Doppler sonogram, showing slow arterial flow in the region of the adnexal branch of the uterine artery. (b) Resected specimen, showing gangrenous ovary

It has been our observation that torsion associated with venous obstruction results in an enlarged but morphologically recognizable ovary[3]. The sonographic findings most probably

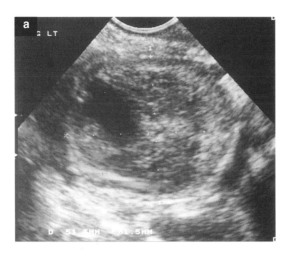

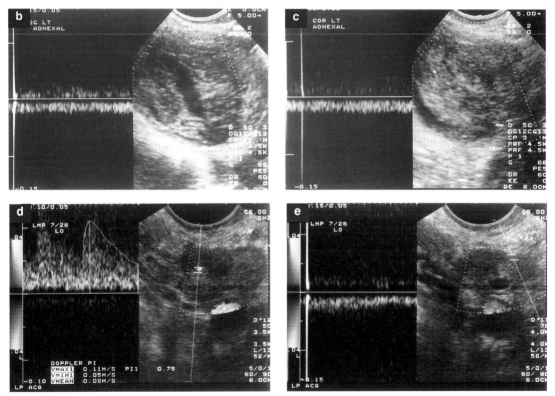

Figure 4 Enlarged ovary found to be viable at surgery in a 28-year-old woman presenting with 2 weeks of intermittent left lower quadrant pain. Transvaginal sonogram (a) demonstrating 5 × 6 cm ovary with an irregular hypoechoic area; triplex transvaginal color Doppler sonograms demonstrating arterial (b) and venous (c) flow within capsular vessels. At surgery, this ovary appeared viable, was untwisted and became perfused as determined by visual inspection. The same patient's left ovary 1 year later, showing normal intraovarian arterial (d) and venous flow (e)

correlate with the presence or absence of intraovarian hemorrhage and chronicity and completeness of the torsion. It is possible that, since the ovary has a dual arterial blood supply, torsion in one arterial system may be compensated by increased flow from blood in the other arterial system. Chronic torsion may be associated with the establishment of collateral arterial and venous flow. As in testicular torsion, repeated episodes might even be associated with a reactive hyperemia.

Rarely, torsion is encountered in normal-sized ovaries[7]. Ovarian and adnexal torsion often produces ovarian enlargement[8]. This may be either diffuse or focal enlargement, related to areas of hemorrhage or the presence of an intraovarian mass[8,9]. When central edema is present, the ovaries may be enlarged with centrally increased echogenicity. Multiple immature follicles may be present along the periphery of the ovary as a result of central ovarian edema[9]. Hemorrhage within the ovary usually produces hypoechoic areas that either are homogeneous or contain delicate linear and punctate echogenicities arising from fibrin strands.

Doppler findings in adnexal torsion relate to the completeness and chronicity of the torsion[3,10,11] (Figures 3–12). Initially, venous flow is reduced, since it has lower intrinsic pressure than the arterial side of the ovarian circulation. Intraovarian arterial signals show high impedance and in extreme cases reversed diastolic flow. Arterial flow is typically maintained in the 'feeding vessels' such as the main ovarian artery and adnexal branch of the uterine artery; occasionally, torsion can be observed in the vascular pedicle itself (Figure 13)[12].

Isolated tubal torsion usually produces enlargement of the tube as identified by its fusiform shape and hypoechoic center[13]. Thickening of the tubal wall may be observed in some cases of adnexal torsion (Figures 11 and 12)[14,15]. Absent or reversed diastolic flow is usually associated with gangrenous changes in the wall. The fusiform mass representing the twisted tube can be seen as separate from the normal ovary.

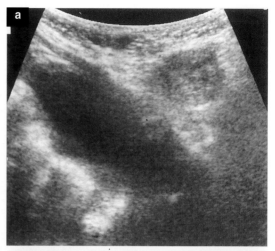
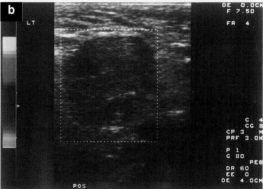
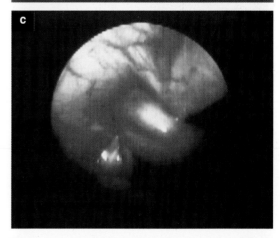

Figure 5 Herniated, twisted ovary in a 5-month-old infant. (a) Transabdominal sonogram, showing mildly enlarged ovary anterior and inferior to bladder. (b) Transabdominal color Doppler sonogram, showing no flow within the ovary. (c) Laparoscopic finding of adnexa herniated through inguinal ring

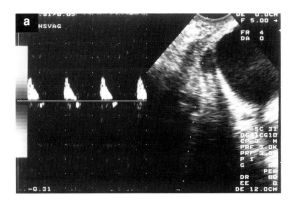

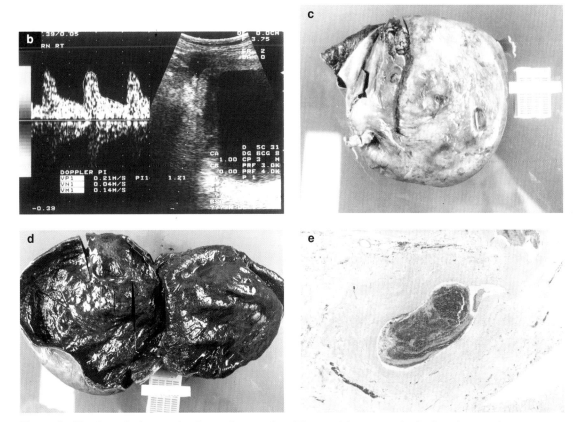

Figure 6 Torsion of a hemorrhagic ovarian cyst in a 50-year-old woman who had undergone hysterectomy 8 years previously. She presented with a 3-day history of right lower quadrant and flank pain. (a) Transvaginal color Doppler sonogram, showing absent diastolic flow in adnexal branch of uterine artery. The ovary contained a hemorrhagic mass. (b) Transvaginal color Doppler sonogram, showing an area of intermediate impedance to flow, adjacent to the hemorrhagic mass. (c) Excised specimen, showing twisted vascular pedicle, but perfused tube. (d) Opened specimen, showing areas of hemorrhage. (e) Low-power photomicrograph, showing thrombus within an intraovarian vein

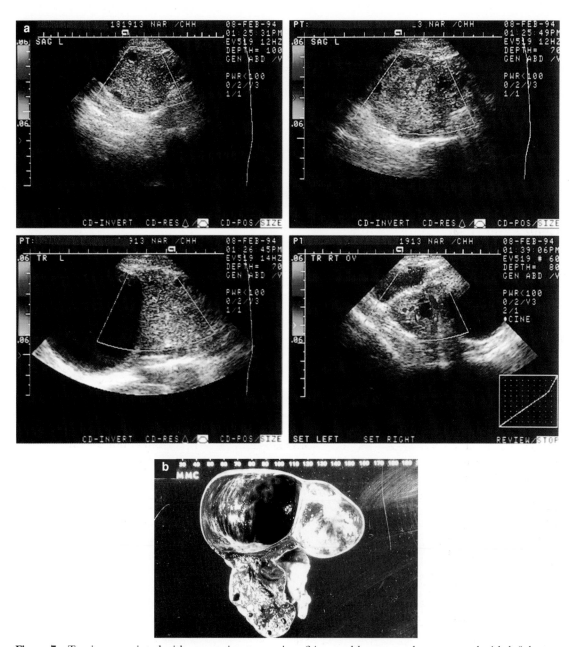

Figure 7 Torsion associated with an ovarian tumor in a 34-year-old woman who presented with left lower quadrant pain for several days. She had a similar episode 5 months previously. (Courtesy of Mary Warner, MD). (a) Composite transvaginal color Doppler sonogram, showing enlarged left ovary demonstrating intraovarian flow adjacent to cystic mass. The right ovary (bottom right) also had intraovarian flow surrounding a corpus luteum. (b) Opened specimen, showing hemorrhagic ovarian mass arising from the left ovary, which also contained several immature follicles and one corpus luteum

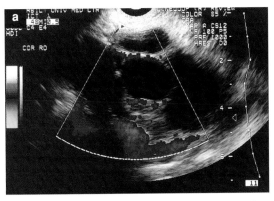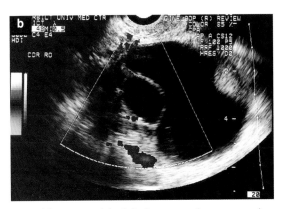

Figure 8 Twisted functional corpus luteum cyst in a 21-year-old woman with right lower quadrant worsening over 1 day. (a) Initial amplitude-color Doppler sonography showed flow within the wall of this septated cyst; 24 h later (b), reduced flow was apparent in this twisted ovarian cyst

Color Doppler sonography findings: sensitivity and specificity

The diagnosis of adnexal torsion by color Doppler sonography is not as simple as documentation of the presence or absence of flow[3,10]. Rather, the color Doppler sonography findings are related to the chronicity and completeness of torsion as well as to its cause. In chronic torsion, there may be arterial collateralization of flow, but in acute torsion, the first and only finding may be lack of venous flow within the ovary. Recent experimental data suggest that chronic torsion may be associated with non-pulsatile arterial waveforms that mimic venous waveforms[16]. Another study reports CDS visualization of the twisted vascular pedicle[17].

We have reviewed 14 cases of documented torsion and have found that the presence of central venous flow is usually associated with a viable (non-gangrenous) adnexa[3]. With torsion, arterial flow may be seen in the capsular branches but is usually absent in the intraovarian branches (Figure 3). One CDS finding that may help distinguish viable from non-viable ovaries is the presence of central venous flow in potentially viable twisted ovaries[3]. CDS may help monitor the presence of flow in ovaries that have undergone surgical detorsion.

In torsion related to areas of hemorrhage or a mass, absent flow is usually present in the area of the mass, whereas flow may be present within the ovary itself (Figure 6). In particular, focal areas of corpus luteum formation may still demonstrate significant flow, whereas areas around the mass are avascular (Figure 7). Tubal torsion may be recognized by a fusiform structure created by the hydrosalpinx[17]. Flow within the thickened wall may be seen, but absent or reversed diastolic flow on waveform analysis is sometimes demonstrated[17] (Figure 11).

There have been only a few reports of color Doppler sonography findings in documented adnexal torsion[3,10,11]. Fortunately, this is a relatively rare condition, even though as sonologists and sonographers we are frequently requested to exclude this possibility, not uncommonly in the middle of the night.

As is illustrated in this chapter, the flow distribution pattern depicted by color Doppler sonography probably has greater diagnostic significance than waveform analysis for assessing the presence or absence of flow within the ovary. Twisted ovaries in young girls may demonstrate flow in the early stages of the disorder. In a report of 14 cases, flow was found in approximately 40%[18]. Similarly, in a report of four cases of proven torsion, flow was documented in one that was successfully treated by untwisting the pedicle[19]. There still exists the caveat that detorsion of the vessels of a twisted ovary containing clot may precipitate pulmonary embolization[20,21].

The improved delineation of flow by power color Doppler may improve the detection of

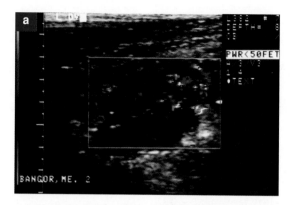

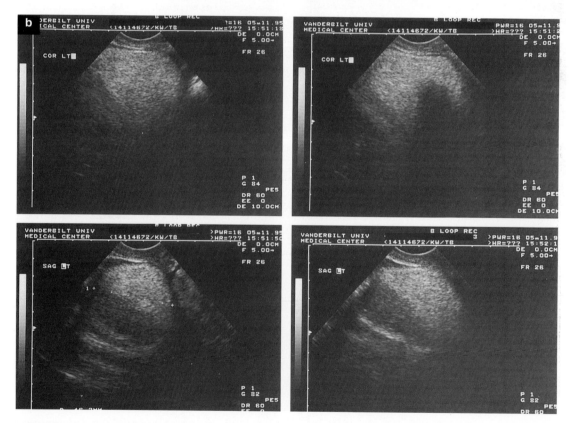

Figure 9 Torsion during pregnancy. (a) Enlarged ovary in a patient with severe left-sided pain during the mid-trimester. Color Doppler sonography, showing flow to the hilar region of the ovary. At surgery, this was considered to be a viable ovary, since it 'pinked up' after untwisting. (Courtesy of Mary Warner, MD). (b) Composite of initial transvaginal sonograms, showing an echogenic adnexal mass. There was a focal area of shadowing related to a collection of sebum within the dermoid cyst. *Continued*

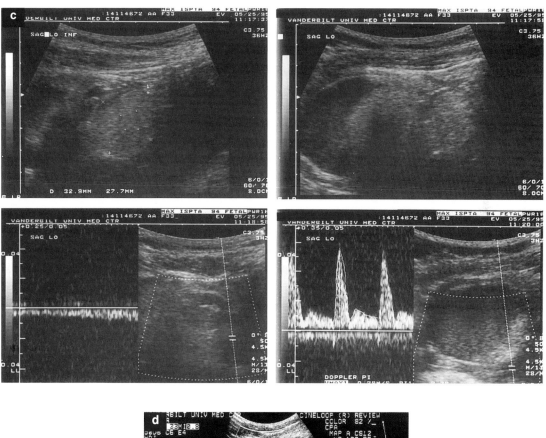

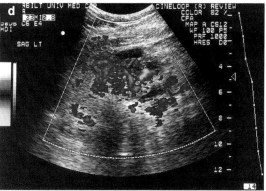

Figure 9 *continued* (c) Composite transvaginal color Doppler sonograms 10 days after detorsion, showing arterial and venous flow. (d) Amplitude color Doppler sonograms, showing flow in the detorsed ovary

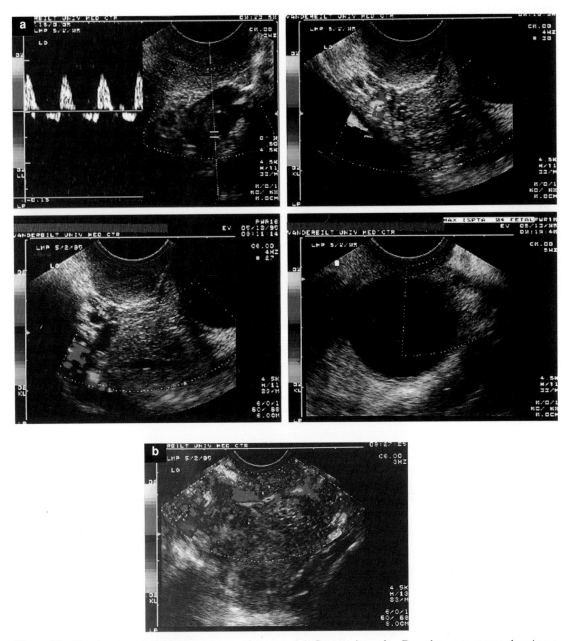

Figure 10 Torsion associated with a paraovarian cyst. (a) Composite color Doppler sonograms showing a paraovarian cyst (lower right) and an enlarged left ovary with reversed flow in an intraovarian arteriole (top left). (b) Color Doppler sonogram of the enlarged, twisted left ovary. The paraovarian cyst was excised and the left ovary was detorsed

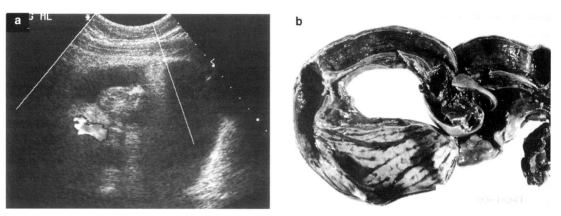

Figure 11 Bilateral tubal torsion in a 35-year-old woman after bilateral tubal ligation. (a) Fusiform mass without flow after tubal ligation. (b) Excised specimen, showing hydrosalpinx and hemorrhagic wall of tube

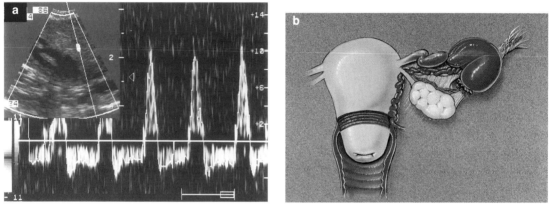

Figure 12 Unilateral tubal torsion in a 53-year-old woman who experienced right lower quadrant pain several days prior to admission. She had undergone bilateral tubal ligation 8 years previously. (a) Transvaginal color Doppler sonogram, showing fusiform mass with thickened wall. There was reversed diastolic flow within the wall of the tube. (b) Diagram of unilateral tubal torsion (drawing by Paul Gross, MS)

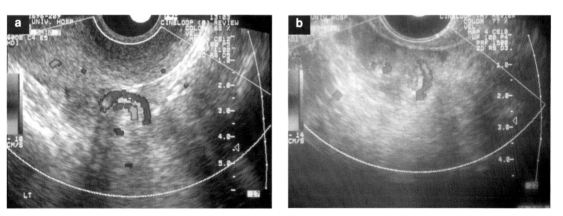

Figure 13 Twisted vascular pedicle (courtesy of Eun Ju Lee, MD, Sawon, Korea). Transvaginal color Doppler sonograms, showing twisted vascular pedicle in a 27-year-old patient (a) with 360° torsion of a teratoma at 9 weeks' gestation; and in a 32-year-old patient (b) with 180° torsion of a right ovarian teratoma

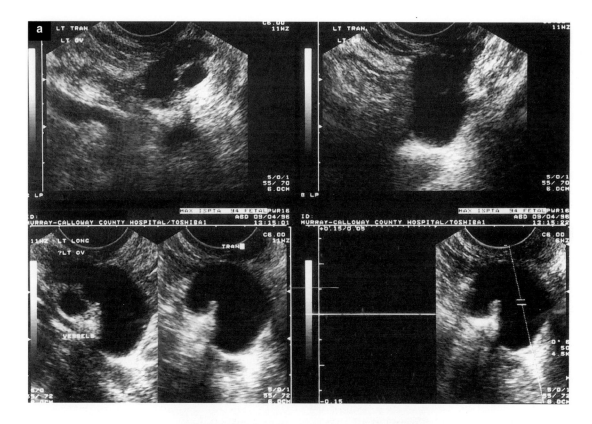

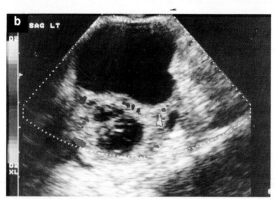

Figure 14 Ovarian remnant syndrome. (a) Composite transvaginal color Doppler sonograms, showing fusiform, a vascular mass in left adnexal area in a patient after oophorectomy. This cyst was aspirated with sonographic guidance. (b) Color Doppler sonogram of cystic mass with areas of hemorrhage in a patient after oophorectomy

focal areas of absent flow with associated with adnexal torsion[22]. Early and prompt diagnosis of adnexal torsion may contribute to conservative surgery, which may spare the ovary from surgical removal.

OVARIAN REMNANT SYNDROME

Ovarian remnant syndrome is an uncommon complication of difficult bilateral oophorectomy. The pain associated with the retained ovarian tissue is usually described as constant, dull,

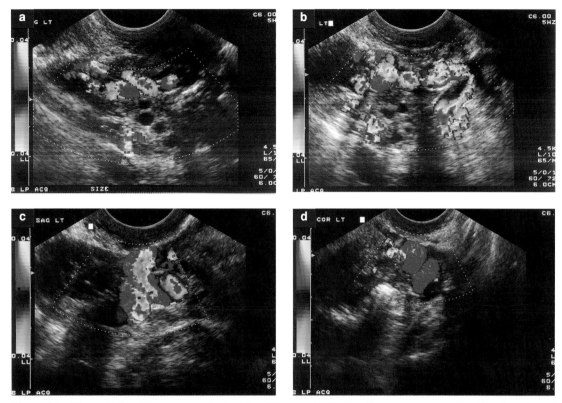

Figure 15 Distended pelvic (parauterine) veins. Transvaginal color Doppler sonography showing dilated uterine veins adjacent to the left ovary as seen in the long (a) and short (b) axis in a patient who was symptomatic; and showing distended parauterine veins in the long (c) and short (d) axis in an asymptomatic woman

diffuse or non-radiating, as well as being localized to the mass. It is theorized that this syndrome can arise from remnants of ovarian cortex that are left behind after oophorectomy. These remnants can become cystic and hemorrhagic[23].

On transvaginal sonography, the remnant tissue can appear as cystic, hemorrhagic masses near the ovarian fossae (Figure 14). Low-impedance flow can be seen in these, owing to the presence of corpora lutea. The hemorrhagic corpus luteum may in turn exert extrinsic pressure on the distal ureter, causing partial ureteric obstruction.

PELVIC CONGESTION SYNDROME

Pelvic congestion syndrome can be the source of chronic pelvic pain. On transvaginal CDS, it is manifested by dilated arcuate, ovarian and uterine veins, which contain slow 'to and fro'

flow in dilated venous structures (Figure 15). The veins become even more distended on the Valsalva maneuver. There is significant controversy as to the clinical importance of these findings, since some patients with these findings will not experience significant pelvic pain (Figure 16).

In order to obtain better understanding of the relationship between this syndrome and impaired venous return from the pelvis, it is important to appreciate certain anatomical features which may predispose to this condition. The right ovarian vein drains directly into the inferior vena cava, whereas the left empties into the left renal vein. The ovarian vein usually contains several valves, which can become incompetent. Dilatation of the vein occurs during pregnancy, owing to increased flow, and the diameter of the ovarian vein is usually less than 5 mm. Ovarian vein thrombosis may result in

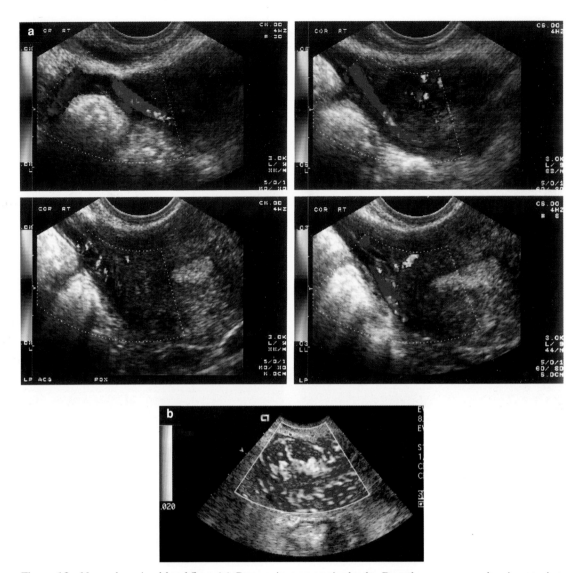

Figure 16 Normal uterine blood flow. (a) Composite transvaginal color Doppler sonogram, showing uterine vein extending into the myometrium as arcuate vein and arcuate arteries in between the outer and middle layers of myometrium. (b) Amplitude color Doppler sonogram, showing arcuate radial and spiral vessels

reduced venous return, further predisposing the patient to edema of the ovarian stroma.

Venous drainage from the adnexal structures also includes the uterine plexus, which drains the parametrium and the ovarian veins, which drain the ovarian blood flow into the internal iliac vein[24]. The uterine and vaginal plexus drain via the uterine veins, usually three on each side, and these form at the level of the cervix and run to the lateral pelvic wall and into the internal iliac vein. The fundal part of the uterine plexus drains partially into the uterine veins and partially into the ovarian venous plexus.

It has been our experience that ovarian and uterine veins may be somewhat dilated in multiparous rather than in nulliparous women, particularly in those with retroflexed uteri. It may be postulated that this position of the uterus may contribute to a diminution in venous return. It can further be hypothesized that decreased venous return from the ovary may contribute to ovarian edema and, therefore,

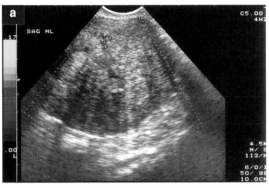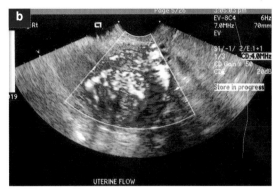

Figure 17 Abnormal uterine flow. Amplitude color Doppler sonography of adenomyosis (a) No significant increased flow as seen within the abnormal myometrium; and (b) showing displaced vessels surrounding an intramural fibroid

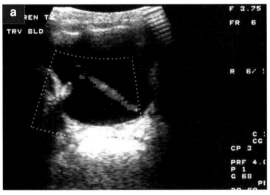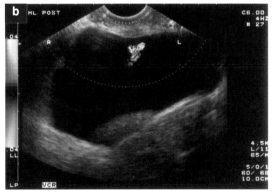

Figure 18 Ureteral jets. (a) Transabdominal color Doppler sonogram, showing a ureteral jet arising from the left ureterovesicular orifice. (b) Transvaginal color Doppler sonogram, showing a ureteral jet arising from the left ureteric orifice

eventually make the ovary more susceptible to torsion.

Transvaginal color Doppler sonography demonstrates distended venous structures in the adnexa[25] (Figure 15). The diameter of these venous structures is usually greater than 3–4 mm and the flow within them is slow (< 3 cm/s) and sometimes lacks respiratory variation or periodicity.

The correlation of these sonographic findings with the clinical syndrome associated with pelvic congestion has been described[25–27]. This syndrome is characterized by pain produced with adnexal palpation, dysmenorrhea, dysfunctional bleeding and/or painful intercourse. Before the development of transvaginal CDS, the diagnosis was made on phlebography by direct injection into the myometrium.

Treatment is directed towards alleviation of the anatomical situation associated with pelvic congestion, namely surgical correction of uterine retroflexion. Some have treated this condition with embolization of the ovarian veins or medically with non-steroidal analgesics[28]. Antithrombotic drugs have also been used, with variable success. For further information, the reader is referred to several articles which describe the syndrome and its treatment in greater detail[25–28].

MISCELLANEOUS CAUSES OF PELVIC PAIN SEEN WITH CDS

TVS and transvaginal CDS can be used to diagnosis several causes of pelvic pain that are relatively rare, such as distal ureteral calculi,

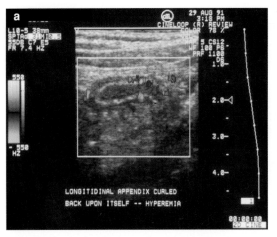
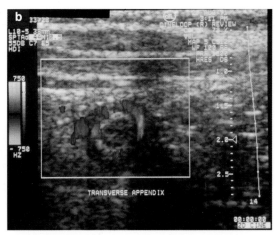

Figure 19 Transabdominal color Doppler sonography of appendicitis. (a) A fusiform mass is depicted at McBurney's point, with hyperemia within the wall, representing an inflamed appendix. (b) Same as (a), seen on short axis

appendicitis and other bowel disorders and adenomyosis (Figures 16–19). Adenomyosis is a condition usually associated with endometriosis, in which endometrial tissue is implanted within the myometrium as well as within the endometrium. The endometrial implants may hemorrhage and produce pain during menses. On CDS, myometrial areas can contain punctate areas of flow as opposed to fibroids, which are typically supplied by circumferentially arranged vessels (Figure 17)[28].

The distal ureter can be evaluated by TVS[29]. Calculi within a distended ureter near the ureterovesicle junction can be determined by looking for the urine jet arising from the ureteral orifice (Figure 18).

Appendicitis can be recognized by either transabdominal sonography (TAS) or TVS by an abnormally thickened (> 3 mm single wall thickness) bowel loop in the right lower quadrant (Figure 19). Although the condition is usually best depicted by the transabdominal approach, the proximity of bowel within the cul-de-sac to the TVS probe may allow diagnosis by this approach[30]. Even though the signs of appendicitis are usually non-specific, one may encounter patients with pain that does not allow them to keep their leg down. This is called the 'psoas' sign. The reader is referred to an excellent review which describes the complete spectrum of clinical findings in appendicitis[31].

Ischemic bowel appears as an abnormally thickened aperistaltic loop. CDS may show absent flow the bowel wall[32]. Certain inflammatory diseases such as Crohn's disease can be associated with increased flow within the bowel wall.

Adhesions secondary to previous surgery may be seen if fluid is on either side of them. Otherwise, adhesive disease may be implied if the uterus and ovaries do not move independently when the probe is introduced ('sliding organ sign').

SUMMARY

Transvaginal CDS has an important role in the evaluation of women with pelvic pain, primarily in establishing or excluding adnexal torsion, which requires immediate surgical intervention. CDS findings reflect the completeness and chronicity of torsion, ranging from absent intraovarian venous flow to reversed diastolic flow within the intraovarian arterioles. CDS can also be helpful in the diagnosis of ovarian remnant syndrome and pelvic congestion syndrome, as well as other non-gynecological causes of pelvic pain such as appendicitis and ureteric obstruction.

References

1. Cunanan, R. G., Courey, N. G. and Lippes, J. (1983). Laparoscopic findings in patients with pelvic pain. *Am. J. Obstet. Gynecol.*, **146**, 589–91

2. Lanig, F. C., Benson, C. B., Disalvo, D. N. *et al.* (1994). Distal ureteral calculi: detection with vaginal US. *Radiology*, **192**, 545–8

3. Fleischer, A., Stein, S., Cullinan, J. and Warner, M. (1995). Color Doppler sonography of adnexal torsion. *J. Ultrasound Med.*, **14**, 523–8

4. Lee, A. R., Kim, K. H., Lee, B. H. *et al.* (1993). Massive edema of the ovary: imaging findings. *Am. J. Roentgenol.*, **161**, 343–4

5. Quillin, S. P. and Siegel, M. J. (1994). Transabdominal color Doppler ultrasonography of the painful adolescent ovary. *J. Ultrasound Med.*, **13**, 549–55

6. Mashiach, S., Bider, D., Moran, O. *et al.* (1990). Adnexal torsion of hyperstimulated ovaries in pregnancies after gonadotropin therapy. *Fertil. Steril.*, **53**, 76–80

7. Worthington-Kirsch, R. L., Raptopoulos, V. and Cohen, I. T. (1986). Sequential bilateral torsion of normal ovaries in a child. *J. Ultrasound Med.*, **5**, 663–4

8. Warner, M. A., Fleischer, A. C., Edell, S. L. *et al.* (1985). Uterine adnexal torsion: sonographic findings. *Radiology*, **154**, 773–5

9. Graif, M. and Itzchak, Y. (1988). Sonographic evaluation of ovarian torsion in childhood and adolescence. *Am. J. Roentgenol.*, **150**, 647, 647–9

10. Rosado, W. M., Trambert, M. A., Gosink, B. B. *et al.* (1992). Adnexal torsion: diagnosis by using Doppler sonography. *Am. J. Roentgenol.*, **159**, 1251–3

11. Van Voorhis, B. J., Schwaiger, J., Syrop, C. H. *et al.* (1992). Early diagnosis of ovarian torsion by color Doppler ultrasonography. *Fertil. Steril.*, **58**, 215–17

12. Lee, E. (1996). *RSNA Scientific Exhibit*, Chicago, December

13. Kupesic, S. and Kurjak, A. (eds.) (1994). *Ultrasound and the Ovary*. (Carnforth, UK: Parthenon Publishing)

14. Sherer, D. M., Liberto, L., Abramowics, J. S. *et al.* (1991). Endovaginal sonographic features associated with isolated torsion of the Fallopian tube. *J. Ultrasound Med.*, **10**, 107–9

15. Elchalal, U., Caspi, B., Schachter, M. *et al.* (1993). Isolated tubal torsion: clinical and ultrasonographic correlation. *J. Ultrasound Med.*, **2**, 115–17

16. Bude, R. O., Kennelly, M. J., Adler, R. S. and Rubin, J. M. (1995). Preliminary investigations: nonpulsatile arterial waveforms: observations during graded testicular torsion in rats. *Acad. Radiol.*, **2**, 879–82

17. Lee, E. (1996). Diagnosis of torsion of adnexal tumors with color Doppler US: significance of twisted pedicle detection. *RSNA 96 Syllabus*, p. 104

18. Stark, J. E. and Siegel, M. J. (1994). Ovarian torsion in prepubertal and pubertal girls: sonographic findings. *Am. J. Roentgenol.*, **163**, 1479–82

19. Willms, A. B., Schlund, J. F. and Meyer, W. R. (1995). Endovaginal Doppler ultrasound in ovarian torsion: a case series. *Ultrasound Obstet. Gynecol.*, **5**, 129–32

20. Gordon, J. D., Hopkins, K. L., Jeffrey, R. B. and Giudice, L. C. (1994). Adnexal torsion: color Doppler diagnosis and laparoscopic treatment. *Fertil. Steril.*, **61**, 383–5

21. Bider, D., Mashiach, S., Dulitzky, M. *et al.* (1991). Clinical, surgical and pathological findings of adnexal torsion in pregnant and nonpregnant women. *Surg. Gynecol. Obstet.*, **173**, 363–6

22. Fleischer, A. C., Chong, W. K., Cullinan, J. A. and Entman, S. S. (1995). Flow patterns in adnexal torsion as depicted by color Doppler sonography. *Video J. Color Flow Imag.*, **5**, 25–8

23. Lafferty, H. W., Angioli, R., Rudolph, J. and Penalver, M. A, (1994). Ovarian remnant syndrome: experience at Jackson Memorial Hospital, University of Miami, 1985 through 1993. *Am. J. Obstet. Gynecol.*, **174**, 641–5

24. Kennedy, A. and Hemingway, A. (1990). Radiology of ovarian varices. *Br. J. Hosp. Med.*, **44**, 38–43

25. Beard, R. W., Reginald, P. W. and Wadsworth, J. (1988). Clinical features of women with chronic lower abdominal pain and pelvic congestion. *Br. J. Obstet. Gynaecol.*, **95**, 153–61

26. Hobbs, J. T. (1990). The pelvic congestion syndrome. *Br. J. Hosp. Med.*, **43**, 200–6

27. Bonilla-Musoles, F. and Ballester, M. (1993). Transvaginal color Doppler in the diagnosis of pelvic congestion syndrome. In Kurjak, A. (ed.) *Transvaginal Color Doppler*, 2nd edn, p.207. (Carnforth, UK: Parthenon Publishing)

28. Sichalaw, M., Yoo, J. and Vogelzang, R. (1994). Transcatheter embolotherapy for treatment of pelvic congestion syndrome. *Obstet. Gynecol.*, **83**, 892–6

29. Laing, F. C., Benson, C. B., DiSalvo, D. *et al.* (1994). Distal ureteral calculi: detection with vaginal US. *Radiology*, **192**, 545–8

30. Puylaert, J. (1994). TVS for Dx of appendicitis. Letter to Editor. *Am. J. Roentgenol.*, **163**, 746

31. Wagner, J. M., McKinney, W. P. and Carpenter, J. L. (1996). Does this patient have appendicitis? *J. Am. Med. Assoc.*, **276**, 1589–94

32. Jeffery, R., Sommer, F. and Debotcu, J. (1994). Color Doppler sonography of focal gastrointestinal lesions: initial clinical experience. *J. Ultrasound Med.*, **13**, 473

Doppler assessment of the normal endometrium and benign endometrial disorders

S. Kupesic and A. Kurjak

8

The endometrium appears as an echogenic interface in the central part of the uterus, and transvaginal sonography permits its detailed delineation[1]. Endometrial thickness and texture are highly dependent on the concentration of circulating estrogen and progesterone.

The menstruating portion of the endometrium in normally fertile women is characterized by disintegration and exfoliation of the two functional layers of the endometrium (the compacta and spongiosa)[2]. Only the functionless basal layer, from which regeneration and resurfacing of the endometrium occur, remains intact. The hormonal deprivation as well as the alterations of the spiral arteriolar system are essential parts of the mechanism. The increased coiling of the spiral arterioles creates circulatory stasis, leading to further tissue ischemia. Vasoconstriction of the spiral arterioles and necrosis of their walls result in bleeding[3]. Anechoic areas which are sometimes visualized indicate endometrial breakdown. Later on, a mixed appearance with anechoic areas (indicating blood) and hyperechoic parts (exfoliated endometrium and clots) can be detected. During the late menstrual phase, the endometrium appears sonographically as a thin, single-line, slightly irregular echogenic interface.

Endometrial thickness of < 5 mm is usually associated with the early follicular phase. The endometrial glands, lined by moderately low columnar cells, are narrowly tubular. Mitotic figures become numerous and blood vessels begin to run upwards from the basal layer towards the surface area of the endometrium, where the capillary network develops. At this stage the endometrium is imaged as a hyperechoic line. Sometimes it is not possible to visualize the endometrial–myometrial junction.

As ovulation approaches, the glands become more numerous and the expected endometrial thickness is about 10 mm. A triple-line endometrium is typical for the periovulatory phase. The hyperechoic echo that represents the endometrial–myometrial junction becomes more prominent and does not produce posterior enhancement. The central echogenic interface probably represents refluxed mucus.

During the secretory phase there is a significant increase of glycogen, acid phosphatase and lipids in the endometrium. It becomes hyperechoic and homogeneous with a loss of the tripleline morphology and surrounding anechoic halo. During this phase of the cycle the ultrasonographic image of the endometrium shows increased echogenicity with respect to the myometrium. The interface of the myometrium with the endometrium is still visible as a hypoechoic zone. Maximum echogenicity is seen in the midluteal phase, when the endometrium appears homogeneously hyperechoic. Posterior enhancement is a sonographic characteristic of this phase. By using transvaginal color and pulsed Doppler sonography (TVCD) it becomes possible to study the alterations of endometrial perfusion in physiological and pathophysiological conditions.

Increased endometrial vascularity during the menstrual cycle depends on the changes of the uterine, arcuate and radial artery blood flow (Figure 1). Blood flow velocity waveform changes in spiral arteries during the normal ovulatory cycle were described for the first time in 1993 with TVCD[4]. The day before ovulation, the spiral artery blood flow velocity starts increasing, with a resistance index (RI) of 0.54 ± 0.03 (Figure 2). This reaches its nadir of 0.49 ± 0.05 between days 16 and 18. In comparing these patterns with those obtained during the stimulated ovarian cycles it was found that impedance to flow rises during the day before ovulation in the latter cycles. It is possible that induction of ovulation interferes with the uterine response and should be assessed by Doppler studies before embryo transfer (ET). It seems that endometrial perfusion presents a more accurate non-invasive assay of uterine receptivity than uterine artery perfusion alone. Therefore, blood flow velocity waveform changes of spiral arteries may be used to predict the implantation success rate, to reveal unexplained infertility problems and to select patients for correction of endometrial perfusion abnormalities by an appropriate treatment[5] (Table 1).

An interesting study was recently performed by Zaidi and colleagues[6]. The authors evaluated 96 women undergoing *in vitro* fertilization (IVF) treatment on the day of human chorionic gonadotropin (hCG) administration by TVCD. They assessed endometrial thickness, endometrial morphology, the presence or absence of subendometrial or intraendometrial color flow, intraendometrial vascular penetration and subendometrial blood flow velocimetry on the day of hCG administration and related the results to pregnancy rates. The overall pregnancy rate was 32.3% and there was no significant difference between the pregnant and non-pregnant groups with regard to endometrial thickness, subendometrial peak systolic blood flow velocity (V_{max}) or subendometrial pulsatility index (PI). The pregnancy rates based on endometrial morphology were not significantly different, being 17.6%, 33.3% and 35.6% for type A (hyperechoic), type B (isoechoic) and type C

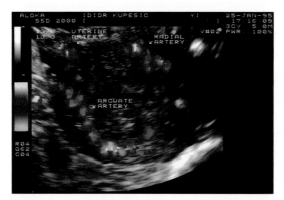

Figure 1 Transvaginal scan of the uterus, demonstrating the uterine vascular network: uterine arteries at the level of cervicocorporeal junction, arcuate arteries encircling the uterus and radial arteries within the myometrial portion

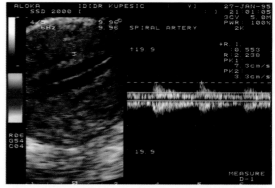

Figure 2 Color signals obtained at the periphery of the multilayered endometrium. Increased blood flow velocity and decreased resistance index (RI = 0.55) occurred during the day of ovulation

Table 1 Spiral artery blood flow during the periovulatory period assessed by transvaginal color Doppler

Day from ovulation	Peak systolic blood flow velocity (cm/s)	Resistance index	Pulsatility index
Spiral artery velocity			
−3	6.21 ± 0.04	0.55 ± 0.02	0.86 ± 0.05
−2	6.02 ± 0.09	0.54 ± 0.03	0.85 ± 0.09
−1	6.32 ± 0.12	0.48 ± 0.04	0.83 ± 0.12
0	6.68 ± 0.68	0.48 ± 0.06	0.84 ± 0.14
+1	7.46 ± 1.31	0.49 ± 0.05	0.72 ± 0.12

(triple-line) endometria, respectively. In eight patients subendometrial color flow and intraendometrial vascularization were not detected. Absence of endometrial blood flow was associated with failure of implantation. Pregnancy rates related to the zones of vascular penetration into the subendometrial and endometrial regions were: 26.7% for Zone 1 (subendometrial zone), 36.4% for Zone 2 (outer hyperechogenic zone) and 37.9% for Zone 3 (inner hypoechogenic zone), and were not significantly different. Of cycles with type A endometrium, 23.5% had absent subendometrial color, which was greater than the frequency of absent color in the type C endometrium.

Our recent study[7] clearly demonstrated that patients with normal endometrial development showed a similar trend of regression for uterine, radial and spiral artery impedance from the follicular to the luteal phase. In contrast, patients with a delayed endometrial pattern and corpus luteum insufficiency were characterized by increased uterine vascular resistance during the luteal phase. Higher impedance values during the periovulatory phase (RI 0.70 ± 0.06, $p < 0.001$), mid-luteal phase (RI 0.72 ± 0.06, $p < 0.001$) and late luteal phase (RI 0.72 ± 0.04, $p < 0.001$) were obtained from the spiral arteries in the group with the luteal phase defect. Since the most significant difference in terms of the RI was obtained for intraovarian and endometrial vessels in patients with corpus luteum insufficiency, one can postulate that color and pulsed Doppler analysis may aid in assessing luteal phase adequacy. Furthermore, this can be used together with hormonal and histological markers of uterine receptivity or even instead of them.

SUBMUCOUS MYOMA

The uterine fibroid is one of the most common tumors of the pelvic viscera in women of reproductive age[8]. Leiomyomas can remain intramural, or they can extend into the uterine lumen to become submucosal or outward to become subserosal or pedunculated. Submucosal myomas are the least common. Clinically,

symptoms such as metrorrhagia, pelvic pain or infertility are usually present in patients with submucous leiomyomas. The existence and severity of symptoms are highly dependent on their number, size and location.

The diagnosis of uterine leiomyoma is based on distortion of the uterine contour, uterine enlargement and textural changes. Since leiomyomas have a varying amount of smooth muscle and connective tissue, these benign tumors also have a variety of sonographic features. Sonographic texture ranges from hypoechoic to echogenic, depending on the amount of smooth muscle and connective tissue.

Sometimes, because of the variety of appearances, leiomyomas may be mistaken for endometrial polyps, blood or mucus. Fedelle and co-workers[9] evaluated the accuracy of transvaginal sonography in detection of small submucous myomas in patients who underwent both transvaginal ultrasound examination and hysteroscopy before hysterectomy. The sensitivity and specificity of transvaginal sonography were similar to those of hysteroscopy in that study. Transvaginal ultrasonography had a sensitivity of 100% and specificity of 94%, while the predictive value of an abnormal ultrasound scan was 81% and that of a normal one was 100%. The sensitivity and specificity of hysteroscopy were 100% and 96%, respectively. The predictive value of an abnormal hysteroscopic finding was 87% and that of a normal result was 100%. Mapping of the uterine leiomyomas is more precise with transvaginal sonography than with hysteroscopy, but the former method can hardly distinguish between a submucous myoma and an endometrial polyp.

The association of leiomyoma with infertility and embryonic fetal wastage is still unknown. It is generally accepted that many women with leiomyomata may conceive and carry pregnancies to term uneventfully. Pregnancy rates ranging from 10 to 89% have been reported in infertile patients who conceived following myomectomy[10]. The origin of infertility associated with leiomyomata is at best uncertain. Several postulated reasons are: a poor nidation site for the conceptus, increased contractility of the uterine musculature, venous alterations in the endometrium and obstruction of the cervix and tubes that may interfere with sperm transport.

Transvaginal sonography with color Doppler imaging facilitates the measurement of blood flow in small vascular branches and increases the reproducibility of the measurements[11] (Table 2).

Kurjak and colleagues[11] evaluated 161 patients: 101 patients with palpable uterine fibroids and 60 healthy volunteers. Waveform analysis was used to quantify the resistance to blood flow in the major arteries supplying identifiable fibroids, as well as in both uterine arteries. Color flow was detected in the border and/or in the center of the tumor (Figure 3). Diastolic flow was always present, usually increased in comparison with uterine artery blood flow. The mean RI of myometrial blood flow was 0.54, and the mean PI was 0.89 (Figure 4). The pathohistological findings were benign uterine tumors in all cases, even when the RI was very low. Decreased RIs were present in cases with necrosis and secondary degenerative and inflammatory changes within the fibroid. Both uterine arteries were visualized, and the Doppler signals were obtained and averaged. In the control group, an RI of 0.84 and PI of 2.52 were noted. Decreased values, such as 0.74 and 1.65 for RI and PI, respectively, were present in patients with uterine fibroids. Blood flow impedance expressed as RI and PI and blood velocity were calculated from the 5th to the 8th day of the cycle. There was a significant difference in the results between patients with palpable uterine fibroids and healthy women attending the clinic for annual checkups. Increased blood flow velocity, and decreased RI and PI in both uterine arteries occurred in patients with uterine fibroids. This study has demonstrated that the vascularization of the tumor is largely dependent on the tumor size and position, as well as on the extent of secondary degenerative changes. Large and laterally positioned fibroids, especially those with necrosis, degenerative and inflammatory changes within myomas, usually show increased diastolic flow and a lower RI ($RI_{min} = 0.35$).

In addition to myoma size, the ultrasound evaluation of a pregnant woman with leiomyoma should include position, location, relationship to the placenta, echogenicity[12] and Doppler evaluation[13]. A statistically significant increased incidence of threatened abortion,

Table 2 Characteristics of blood flow in uterine arteries in patients with palpable (vascularized) uterine fibroids and healthy women

	Controls (n = 60)	Women with vascularized fibroids (n = 81)
Velocity	34.4 ± 12.25	47.08 ± 18.46
RI	0.84 ± 0.09	0.74 ± 0.09
PI	2.52 ± 0.87	1.65 ± 0.49

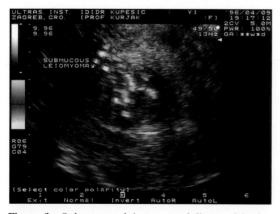

Figure 3 Submucous leiomyoma delineated by increased vascularity. Color Doppler signals demonstrate rich vascular supply at the base of the leiomyoma pedicle

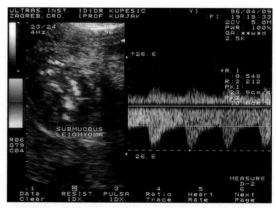

Figure 4 The same patient as in Figure 3. Waveform analysis (right) indicates moderate vascular impedance (RI = 0.55)

preterm delivery, abruptio placentae and pelvic pain was observed in patients with uterine myomas ($p < 0.001$)[12]. Abruptio placentae was particularly evident in women with myoma volumes greater than 200 cm^3, submucosal location or superimposition of the placenta.

Kessler and associates[13] have shown that a conventional ultrasound scan cannot distinguish a local thickening of the uterine wall caused by contraction from a myoma. In such cases repeated scans approximately 30 min later differentiated resolved contractions from myomas. The authors examined ten patients with B-mode and color Doppler ultrasonography. In five patients with myoma they obtained splaying of the vessels around the mass, whereas in five patients with contractions there was no vessel displacement in the area of the local myometrial thickening. Therefore, the use of color Doppler may obviate a prolonged ultrasound examination in questionable cases.

Reinsch and colleagues[14] have examined the effects of RU 486 and leuprolide acetate on uterine artery blood flow and uterine volume in patients with uterine leiomyoma. Patients receiving RU 486 showed a progressive increase in uterine artery RI; uterine artery flow decreased by 40%. Patients receiving leuprolide acetate have shown a 21% decrease in uterine artery perfusion. Simultaneously, the authors noted a significant decrease in uterine volume compared with pretreatment in both groups at 3 months. It was postulated that a decrease in uterine artery blood flow provided a mechanism for the decrease in uterine size and the decrease in uterine blood loss at the time of surgery or hysteroscopy.

ENDOMETRIAL POLYPS

The importance of endometrial polyps lies in the fact that marked reduction in blood flow impedance noted on the periphery and/or within the endometrial polyps may lead an inexperienced ultrasonographer to a false-positive diagnosis of endometrial malignancy. Endometrial polyps are best imaged during the early proliferative phase of the menstrual cycle or after injection of the 'negative' contrast into the uterine cavity.

Endometrial polyps develop as solitary or multiple soft, sessile and penduculated tumors often composed of hyperplastic endometrium[15,16]. Approximately two-thirds contain no functional endometrium, and they often display a microscopic picture of cystic hyperplasia. The vascularization of endometrial polyps is supported by already existing vessels originating from terminal branches of the uterine arteries. It is possible to identify flow in regularly separated vessels and analyze the velocity of blood flow through them (Table 3, Figure 5). The diastolic flow is always present, and RI is usually higher than 0.45[15,17] (Figure 6). In patients with necrotic and inflamed polyps, the RI tends to decrease ($RI_{min} = 0.37$). Polypoid structures can be visualized in infertile patients on gonadotropin releasing hormone (GnRH) therapy, but these structures usually disappear in the next cycle if the IVF procedure was unsuccessful.

Table 3 Vascularization of benign uterine lesions

	n	RI
Submucous myoma	38	0.54 ± 0.06
Adenomyosis	62	0.57 ± 0.08
Endometritis	28	0.50 ± 0.06
Incomplete abortion	31	0.41 ± 0.02
Endometrial polyp	46	> 0.45

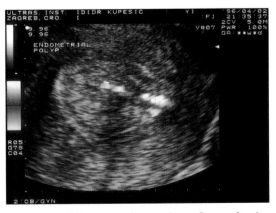

Figure 5 Oblique scan in a patient of reproductive age demonstrating a focal area of increased echogenicity typical of endometrial polyp. Regularly separated vessels are easily visualized

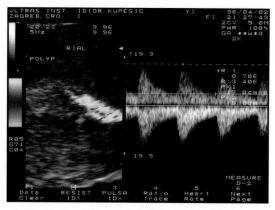

Figure 6 In the same patient as in Figure 5, waveform analysis (right) shows high-resistance blood flow (RI = 0.71) typical of an endometrial polyp

Tamoxifen

Tamoxifen is a non-steroidal antiestrogen that is widely used in the hormonal therapy of breast cancer. However, it has been proposed that tamoxifen can also be given to apparently healthy women at increased risk of breast cancer. The weak estrogen-like effect that tamoxifen has on endometrium is a cause of great concern. Patients using tamoxifen should therefore be monitored at regular intervals, since several studies have described endometrial cancer cases associated with this therapy. A wide spectrum of pathological uterine findings has been described in association with long-term tamoxifen therapy at a dose of 20 mg/day[18]. These findings include epithelial metaplasia, simple and atypical hyperplasia, endometrial polyps and endometrial carcinoma[19]. Endometrial changes are characterized sonographically by abnormal endometrial thickening and heterogeneous hyperechogenicity with multiple, small cystic structures. Goldstein has also described subendometrial cysts, probably representing re-activated adenomyomas[20]. At least three studies have indicated that tamoxifen treatment in postmenopausal breast cancer patients is associated with a high incidence of endometrial polyps[21-23]. Achiron and co-workers[22] found that a peculiar endometrial honeycomb appearance manifested on gray-scale transvaginal sonography occurred in

44% of this population, and was associated with the same high incidence (40%) of endometrial polyps.

However, two large studies on tamoxifen therapy in postmenopausal women failed to correlate endometrial thickness of more than 5 mm with pathological results[24,25].

The effect of tamoxifen on endometrial blood flow has been less evaluated. Achiron and colleagues[26] described blood flow changes in the endometrial and subendometrial regions. In asymptomatic postmenopausal patients receiving tamoxifen whose endometrial thickness was < 5 mm an increase was reported in endometrial blood flow with significant reduction of the RI compared to untreated, control menopausal women. Another study by the same group[19] found that women with thick endometrium, and particularly those with endometrial polyps, presented a significantly lower RI (mean 0.39 vs. 0.79) compared to those with thin endometrium. The RI values returned to normal following resection of the endometrial polyps, thus supporting a benign transitory effect of long-term tamoxifen therapy on the endometrium.

Huang and associates[27] described two cases of endometrial adenofibroma in patients on tamoxifen therapy. Adenofibroma is a rare, benign, mixed mesodermal tumor. The sonographic characteristics of adenofibroma are different from those of endometrial polyp, endometrial hyperplasia and endometrial carcinoma. The characteristic swollen villi that produce a snowstorm-like sonographic image in gestational trophoblastic disease resemble the findings of adenofibroma. However, a differential diagnosis can be made using transvaginal color and pulsed Doppler. Lucunae filled with turbulent blood flow are observed in patients with gestational trophoblastic disease, whereas higher vascular impedance suggests endometrial adenofibroma.

ENDOMETRIAL HYPERPLASIA

The endometrial echo in postmenopausal women is generally no more than a thin linear echo usually 1–3 mm in thickness. Abnormal endometrial thickness may be detected in some benign uterine conditions such as endometrial hyperplasia. Endometrial thickness of > 14 mm in premenopausal and > 5 mm in postmenopausal women should be an indicator for further investigation[15]. The peak incidence of adenomatous hyperplasia is between 40 and 50 years of age. Morphology itself cannot be used to discriminate benign from malignant conditions, since the problem of differentiating endometrial hyperplasia from carcinoma is still unsolved by B-mode transvaginal sonography alone.

Endometrial hyperplasia and endometrial carcinoma are angiogenic, and should therefore

be detected by sensitive Doppler units. Color and pulsed Doppler features serve as additional discriminative criteria for more accurate diagnosis of endometrial pathology[16,17]. The peripheral distribution of the regularly separated vessels is typical of endometrial hyperplasia (Figure 7). Color flow and pulsed Doppler signals are usually obtained from the border of the hyperplastic endometrium (Table 3). A significant difference has been found in terms of the RI value between endometrial malignancy (mean RI = 0.42) and endometrial hyperplasia (mean RI = 0.50)[28] (Figures 8 and 9). Some clinicians have begun to utilize sonographic and Doppler evaluation to decide which patients should undergo biopsy and which patients can simply be followed. This can be particularly useful in elderly patients in poor medical condition, as well as in patients with stenotic cervical os.

The study of Gredmark and co-workers[29] has shown that the histopathological finding of endometrial adenomatous hyperplasia or cancer occurred in about 15% of postmenopausal women with bleeding, and the endometrium was atrophic in 50%. This finding implies that ultrasound and Doppler examinations should be included in the evaluation of postmenopausal bleeding to avoid endometrial biopsy of atrophic endometrium and/or coincidentally to detect ovarian pathology.

Kurjak and colleagues[30] reported that transvaginal color and pulsed Doppler is a noninvasive procedure that can detect endometrial

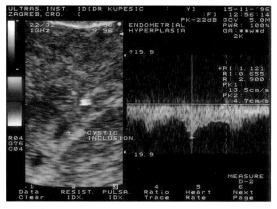

Figure 7 Short-axis view in a postmenopausal patient showing thickened endometrium (10 mm). Note peripheral distribution of the vessels and moderate resistance index (RI = 0.66), typical of endometrial hyperplasia

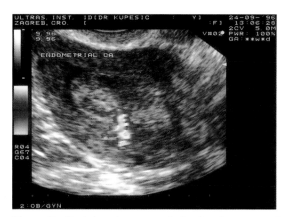

Figure 8 Peripheral neovascularization in a case of endometrial carcinoma demonstrated by color Doppler

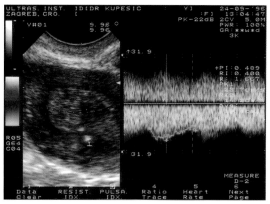

Figure 9 Pulsed Doppler waveform analysis, revealing low resistance index (RI = 0.40), typical of endometrial carcinoma

carcinoma even in asymptomatic women and may be used as a screening procedure. However, Sheth and co-workers[31] reported some overlap between the PI and RI of benign and malignant endometrial lesions. Endometrial arterial flow was seen in 23 out of 36 (64%) proven benign endometrial lesions. The mean RI was 0.48 ± 0.13 (range 0.27–0.84), and the mean PI was 0.72 ± 0.33 (range 0.31–1.77). Endometrial carcinoma revealed abnormal vascularity in 56% of cases. The mean PI in this group was 0.71 ± 0.32 (range 0.42–1.17), and the mean RI was the same as for benign lesions 0.48 ± 0.15 (range 0.34–0.69).

Chan and associates[32] found transvaginal sonography to be superior to color Doppler imaging in the detection of pathological conditions of the endometrium, but neither method could distinguish benign from malignant lesions. Contrary to these findings Bonilla-Musoles and co-workers[33] estimated a positive correlation between uterine arterial blood flow impedance and likelihood of endometrial malignancy in postmenopausal women.

Since there is a positive correlation between arterial blood flow impedance and number of years from menopause[34], one can estimate the risk of uterine malignancy in postmenopausal patients with decreased vascular resistance.

ADENOMYOSIS

The incidence of adenomyosis has been reported in autopsy data to vary from 10 to 50% and in surgical specimens to vary from 5.6 to 61.5%[35,36]. Adenomyosis of the uterus is a condition in which clusters of endometrial tissue occur deep within the myometrium. This may be localized immediately adjacent to the endometrium, or it may extend through the myometrium, and even penetrate the serosa.

Most patients with adenomyosis have either a normal-sized uterus or non-specific findings of uterine enlargement[37]. A diffusely enlarged uterus with a thickened and 'Swiss cheese' appearance of the myometrium due to areas of hemorrhage and clots within the muscle has been reported as an appearance suggestive of

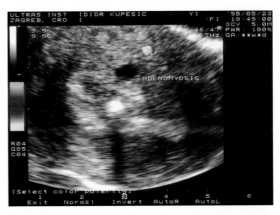

Figure 10 Color flow indicating diffuse blood flow within the thickened 'Swiss cheese' appearance of the myometrium in a patient suffering from dysmenorrhea. Adenomyosis was confirmed by histopathology

adenomyosis[38] (Figure 10). Disordered echogenicity of the middle layer of the myometrium is usually present in severe cases. Sometimes the uterus is generally hypoechoic, while the large cysts are rarely seen. The symptoms generally attributed to adenomyosis include dysmenorrhea, pelvic pain and menometrorrhagia. Significant pain during menstruation is caused by bleeding of the endometrial tissue within the muscle of the uterus. If hysterosalpingography is performed, it may demonstrate contrast medium penetrating the myometrium.

Fedele and colleagues[39] have attempted to clarify the use of endovaginal ultrasound in the diagnosis of diffuse adenomyosis. The sensitivity and specificity were 80% and 74%, respectively. With the use of transvaginal color Doppler and spectral analysis it is possible to study uterine vascularity in this benign condition and to compare it with perfusion in other benign lesions[11,35]. The mean RI of the flow detected within the myometrium covered the value of 0.56, while the RI of the uterine arteries showed a decreased value, such as 0.75, when compared to the values in healthy volunteers (mean RI = 0.87). Some difference between myoma and adenomyoma may be explained by the fact that estrogen receptors are found in higher concentrations in myoma than in the surrounding myometrium. Leiomyomas are therefore responsive to the variations of the luteal hormone[40], but adenomyosis cases demonstrated lack of estrogen and progesterone receptors[41].

Hirai and colleagues[42] examined 44 benign uterine masses and seven uterine malignancies. They used transvaginal color and pulsed Doppler imaging to determine whether this technique is useful for differentiation of adenomyosis from uterine malignancies. For the purpose of this study, the authors also demonstrated a scoring system for diagnosis of adenomyosis. Their scoring system consisted of myometrial thickness, myometrial texture, contour and color Doppler analysis. The RI tended to be lower for uterine malignancies (mean RI = 0.40 ± 0.07) as opposed to adenomyosis (mean RI = 0.57 ± 0.08). The RI for myoma was almost the same as that for adenomyosis (mean RI = 0.57). The maximal velocity (V_{max}) tended to be higher for uterine malignancies than for adenomyosis. The V_{max} for myoma was slightly higher than that for adenomyosis. Their final conclusion was that statistically significant differences exist between adenomyosis and uterine malignancies in both RI and V_{max}. However, no significant difference in RI was noted between adenomyosis and myoma, but a slight difference was observed for V_{max}.

ENDOMETRITIS

In cases of endometritis, increased thickness, echogenicity and vascularity of the endometrium and the inner third of the myometrium can be observed[35]. The waveforms detected from color-coded areas show a moderately high RI (RI > 0.50 ± 0.06) (Table 3). Together with regression of the symptoms, vascularity becomes less prominent, while RI values are elevated.

INCOMPLETE ABORTION

Although the diagnostic capacity of color Doppler ultrasound and its value as a predictor of pregnancy outcome are still unclear, it has markedly reduced the uncertainties in diagnosis of early pregnancy failure[43,44].

Incomplete abortion varies with the stage of embryological development at the time of the demise and the amount of gestational tissue passed. Variable amounts of disorganized echogenic debris, fluid, or both are often present in the endometrial cavity. Transvaginal color Doppler demonstrates rich perfusion of the unexpelled gestational tissue. Abundant color flow is caused by the dilated spiral arteries and venous system, probably in response to the active trophoblastic tissue (Figure 11). Low vascular impedance (RI = 0.41 ± 0.01) can be detected at the endometrial level even without clear viability of the products of conception[44] (Table 3). A mixed endometrial pattern characterized by presence of both hyperechoic and hypoechoic areas remains the mainstay in the diagnosis of incomplete abortion.

DECIDUA

Differentiating between endometrium-derived structures, decidualized tissues, early normal pregnancy and abnormal gestational sacs can be critical to the diagnosis of an amenorrheic patient[45]. When the uterine cavity is empty, shows a decidual reaction or only a weak central fluid ring, a suspicion of ectopic pregnancy must be aroused if the pregnancy test is positive. In a patient with a non-specific complex adnexal mass, transvaginal color Doppler seems to be helpful in demonstrating low-impedance flow on the side of ectopic pregnancy. In contrast to

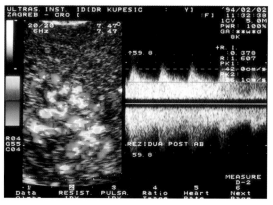

Figure 11 Transvaginal color Doppler demonstrating abundant flow typical of unexpelled gestational tissue (left). Low resistance index (RI = 0.38) detected at the level of the endometrium indicates incomplete abortion

two concentric rings of decidua identified in early intrauterine pregnancy, the decidual ring associated with ectopic pregnancy has only one layer of decidua.

Jurkovic and co-workers[46] compared the vascular signature in these two conditions. They found that blood flow impedance in uterine and spiral arteries, and in corpus luteum blood vessels, showed no significant difference between intrauterine and ectopic pregnancies. The peak-systolic velocity in the uterine arteries was the parameter that precisely reflected increased blood supply to the ectopic pregnancy.

It seems that transvaginal color Doppler has a potential for selection of patients for different treatment options (conservative, non-interventional treatment, minimal invasive surgery or laparotomy).

References

1. Callen, P. W., De Martini, W. J. and Filly, R. A. (1979). The central uterine cavity echo: a useful sign on the ultrasonographic evaluation of the female pelvis. *Radiology*, **131**, 187–90

2. Lawn, A. M. (1974). The ultrastructure of the endometrium. *J. Reprod. Fertil.*, **37**, 239–42

3. Keye, W. R., Yuen, B. H. and Jaffe, R. B. (1973). New concepts in the physiology of the menstrual cycle. *Clin. Endocrinol. Metab.*, **2**, 251–8

4. Kupesic, S. and Kurjak, A. (1993). Uterine and ovarian perfusion during the periovulatory period assessed by transvaginal color Doppler. *Fertil. Steril.*, **60**, 439–43

5. Kupesic, S. (1996). The first three weeks assessed by transvaginal color Doppler. *J. Perinat. Med.*, **24**, 301–17

6. Zaidi, J., Campbell, S., Pittrof, R. and Tan, S. L. (1995). Endometrial thickness, morphology, vascular penetration and velocimetry in predicting implantation in an *in vitro* fertilization program. *Ultrasound Obstet. Gynecol.*, **6**, 191–8

7. Kupesic, S., Kurjak, A., Vujisic, S. and Petrovic, Z. (1997). Luteal phase defect: comparison between Doppler velocimetry, histological and hormonal markers. *Ultrasound Obstet. Gynecol.*, **9**, 1–8

8. Vollenhoven, B. J., Lawrence, A. S. and Healy, D. (1990). Uterine fibroids: a clinical review. *Br. J. Obstet. Gynaecol.*, **97**, 285–98

9. Fedele, L., Bianchi, S., Dorta, M. *et al.* (1991). Transvaginal ultrasonography versus hysteroscopy in the diagnosis of uterine submucous myomas. *Obstet. Gynecol.*, **77**, 745–8

10. Thureck, R. W. (1988). Uterine leiomyomata. In Garcia, C. R., Mastroianni, L., Amelar, R. D. and Dubin, L. (eds.) *Current Therapy of Infertility*, pp. 80–2. (Toronto: B. C. Decker)

11. Kurjak, A., Kupesic-Urek, S. and Miric, D. (1992). The assessment of benign uterine tumor vascularization by transvaginal color Doppler. *Ultrasound Med. Biol.*, **18**, 645–9

12. Exacoustos, C. and Rosati, P. (1993). Ultrasound diagnosis of uterine myomas and complications in pregnancy. *Obstet. Gynecol.*, **82**, 97–101

13. Kessler, A., Mitchell, X. and Goldberg, B. B. (1993). Myoma vs. contraction in pregnancy: differentiation with color Doppler imaging. *J. Clin. Ultrasound*, **21**, 241–4

14. Reinsch, R. C., Murphy, A. A., Morales and Yen, S. S. (1994). The effects of RU 486 and leuprolide acetate on uterine artery blood flow in the fibroid uterus: a prospective randomized study. *Am. J. Obstet. Gynecol.*, **170**, 1623–7

15. Kurjak, A., Kupesic, S., Zalud, I. and Predanic, M. (1995). Transvaginal color Doppler. In Dodson, M. G. (ed.) *Transvaginal Ultrasound*, pp. 325–39 (New York: Churchill Livingstone)

16. Fleischer, A. C., Kepple, D. M. and Entman, S. S. (1991). Transvaginal sonography of uterine disorders. In Timor-Tritsch, I. E. and Rottem, S. (eds.) *Transvaginal Sonography*, 2nd edn, pp. 109–30. (New York: Elsevier)

17. Kurjak, A. and Kupesic, S. (1995). Transvaginal color Doppler and pelvic tumor vascularity: lessons learned and future challenges. *Ultrasound Obstet. Gynecol.*, **6**, 1–15

18. Ismail, S. M. (1994). Pathology of the endometrium treated with tamoxifen. *J. Clin. Pathol.*, **47**, 827–33

19. Achiron, R., Grisaru, D., Golan-Porat, N. and Lipitz, S. (1996). Tamoxifen and the uterus: an old drug tested by new modalities. *Ultrasound Obstet. Gynecol.*, **7**, 374–8

20. Goldstein (1994). *Am. J. Obstet. Gynecol.*

21. Lahti, E., Blanco, G., Kaupilla, A., Apaja-Sarkkinen, M., Taskinen, P. J. and Laatikainen, T. (1993). Endometrial changes in postmenopausal breast cancer patients receiving tamoxifen. *Obstet. Gynecol.*, **81**, 660–4

22. Achiron, R., Lipitz, S., Sivan, E., Goldenberg, M., Horovitz, A., Frenkel, Y. and Maschiah, S.

(1995). Changes mimicking endometrial neoplasia in postmenopausal, tamoxifen-treated women with breast cancer: a transvaginal Doppler study. *Ultrasound Obstet. Gynecol.*, **6**, 116–20

23. Exacoustos, E., Zupi, E., Cangi, B., Chiaretti, M., Arduini, D. and Romanini, C. (1995). Endometrial evaluation in postmenopausal breast cancer patients receiving tamoxifen: an ultrasound, color flow Doppler hysteroscopic and histological study. *Ultrasound Obstet. Gynecol.*, **6**, 435–42

24. Uziely, B., Lewin, A., Brufman, G., Dorembus, D. and Mor-Yosef, S. (1993). The effect of tamoxifen on the endometrium. *Breast Cancer Res. Treat.*, **26**, 101–5

25. Cohen, I., Rosen, D., Trepper, R., Cordova, M., Shai, Y., Altaras, M. M., Yigal, D. and Beyth, Y. (1993). Ultrasonographic evaluation of the endometrium and correlation with endometrial sampling in postmenopausal patients treated with tamoxifen. *J. Ultrasound Med.*, **5**, 275–8

26. Achiron, R., Lipitz, S., Frenkel, Y. and Mashiach, S. (1995). Endometrial blood flow response to estrogen replacement therapy and tamoxifen in asymptomatic postmenopausal women: a transvaginal Doppler study. *Ultrasound Obstet. Gynecol.*, **5**, 411–14

27. Huang, K. T., Chen, C. A., Cheng, W. F., Wu, C. C., Jou, H. J., Hsieh, C. Y., Lin, G. J. and Hsieh, F. J. (1996). Sonographic characteristics of adenofibroma of the endometrium following tamoxifen therapy for breast cancer: two case reports. *Ultrasound Obstet. Gynecol.*, **7**, 363–6

28. Kupesic-Urek, S., Shalan, H. and Kurjak, A. (1993). Early detection of endometrial cancer by transvaginal color Doppler. *EUROBS*, **49**, 46–9

29. Gredmark, T., Huint, S., Havel, G. and Mattsson, L. A. (1995). Histopathological findings in women with postmenopausal bleeding. *Br. J. Obstet. Gynaecol.*, **102**, 133–6

30. Kurjak, A., Shalan, H., Kupesic, S., Kosuta, D., Sosic, A., Benic, S., Ilijas, M., Jukic, S. and Predanic, M. (1994). An attempt to screen asymptomatic women for ovarian and endometrial cancer with transvaginal color and pulsed Doppler sonography. *J. Ultrasound Med.*, **13**, 295–301

31. Sheth, S., Hamper, V. M., McCollum, M. E., Caskey, C. I., Rosenshein, N. B. and Khurman, R. J. (1995). Endometrial blood flow analysis in postmenopausal women: can it help differentiate benign from malignant causes of endometrial thickening. *Radiology*, **195**, 661–5

32. Chan, F. Y., Chau, M. T., Pun, T. C., Lam, C., Ngan, H. Y., Leong, L. and Wong, R. L. (1994). Limitation of transvaginal sonography and color Doppler imaging in the differentiation of endometrial carcinoma from benign lesions. *J. Ultrasound Med.*, **13**, 623–8

33. Bonilla-Musoles, F., Marti, M. C., Ballester, M. J., Raga, F. and Osborne, N. G. (1995). Normal uterine arterial blood flow in postmenopausal women assessed by transvaginal color Doppler ultrasonography. *J. Ultrasound Med.*, **14**, 491–4

34. Kurjak, A. and Kupesic, S. (1995). Ovarian senescence and its significance on uterine and ovarian perfusion. *Fertil. Steril.*, **3**, 532–7

35. Kurjak, A. and Zalud, I. (1991). The characterization of uterine tumors by transvaginal color Doppler. *Ultrasound Obstet. Gynecol.*, **1**, 50–2

36. Seidler, D., Laing, F. C., Jeffrey, R. B. Jr and Wing, V. W. (1987). Uterine adenomyosis – a difficult sonographic diagnosis. *J. Ultrasound Med.*, **6**, 345–8

37. Bohlman, M. E., Ensor, R. E. and Sanders, R. C. (1987). Sonographic findings in adenomyosis of the uterus. *Am. J. Radiol.*, **184**, 765–6

38. Siedler, D., Lang, F. C., Jeffrey, R. B. and Wing, V. W. (1987). Uterine adenomyosis – a difficult sonographic diagnosis. *J. Ultrasound Med.*, **6**, 345–9

39. Fedele, I., Bianchi, S., Dorta, *et al.* (1992). Transvaginal ultrasonography in the diagnosis of diffuse adenomyosis. *Fertil. Steril.*, **58**, 94

40. Soules, M. R. and McCarty, K. S. Jr (1982). Leiomyoma: steroid receptor content. Variation within normal menstrual cycles. *Am. J. Obstet. Gynecol.*, **143**, 6–11

41. Droegmueller, E. (1992). Endometriosis and adenomyosis. In Manning, S., Steinborn, E. and Salway, J. (eds.) *Comprehensive Gynecology*, pp. 545–76 (St Louis: Mosby Year Book)

42. Hirai, M., Shibata, K., Sagai, H., Sekiya, S. and Goldberg, B. B. (1995). Transvaginal pulsed and color Doppler sonography for the evaluation of adenomyosis. *J. Ultrasound Med.*, **14**, 529–32

43. Stabile, I., Grudzinkas, J. and Campbell, S. (1990). Doppler ultrasonographic evaluation of abnormal pregnancies in the first trimester. *J. Clin. Ultrasound*, **18**, 497–501

44. Jauniaux, E., Jurkovic, D. and Campbell, S. (1991). *In vivo* investigation of the anatomy and the physiology of early human placental circulations. *Ultrasound Obstet. Gynecol.*, **1**, 435–45

45. Dodson, M. G. and Gast, M. (1995). Early pregnancy. In Dodson, M. G. (ed.) *Transvaginal Ultrasound*, pp. 187–217. (New York: Churchill Livingstone)

46. Jurkovic, D., Bourne, T., Jauniaux, E., Campbell, S. and Collins, P. W. (1992). Transvaginal color Doppler study of blood flow in ectopic pregnancy. *Fertil. Steril.*, **57**, 68–73

Tumor angiogenesis in ovarian and endometrial cancer: sonographic depiction and clinical implications

9

A. C. Fleischer

INTRODUCTION

Sonographic depiction of blood flow within the uterus and ovary has significant clinical applications. Besides reflecting changes in the physiological and endocrinological milieu, sonographic depiction of changes in vascularity can enable early detection of ovarian or endometrial malignancy[1,2]. In this chapter, the fundamental principles of tumor angiogenesis and its sonographic depiction in ovarian and endometrial cancers are discussed and illustrated.

TUMOR ANGIOGENESIS: FUNDAMENTAL PRINCIPLES

Tumor angiogenesis differs from regulated angiogenesis in wound healing or the formation of placenta or corpus luteum in that, in the latter conditions, vessel growth is orderly and controlled. Tumor angiogenesis is disorderly and uncontrolled. Tumor vessels arise from the host vasculature by promoting endothelial growth by elaboration of vasogenic growth factors. These substances stimulate vessel budding from the host vasculature. The tumor vessels contain numerous arteriovenous shunts and vessels that lack a muscular media, which imparts a certain vascular tone to normal arterioles. The vascular network of tumor contains vessels that have numerous segments of stenoses and dilatation. Since the vessels that supply the tumor typically arise from the venous supply, which has lower pressure, there is an overall increase in flow, especially in the diastolic phase. Tumor vessels are also 'leaky', owing to poor perivascular support. These microvascular changes can be recognized on Doppler interrogation as vessels with low-impedance waveform patterns and relatively high velocities, due to areas of vessel narrowing. With the recent technological advances such as amplitude and phase aberration depiction, and the combination of contrast enhancement with harmonic imaging, some of these features are now also becoming apparent on color Doppler studies.

MICROVESSEL DENSITY: CLINICAL IMPLICATIONS

The correlation of tumor microvessel density seen on histology and metastatic potential has been reported for a variety of tumors including breast, prostate, cervical, endometrial and ovarian cancers[3]. In fact, some believe that intratumor microvessel density may be a better predictor of disease-free survival than stage, grade and tumor type.

Recent reports have shown a correlation between microvessel density in ovarian and endometrial cancers and likelihood of recurrence[4,5]. In a series of patients with advanced ovarian cancer, low vessel counts were associated with longer survival[4]. This study concluded that analysis of neovascularization in advanced ovarian cancer may be a useful prognostic factor. In a group of patients with endometrial cancer, those with a low capillary density had a mean survival time of 123 months vs. 75 months for those with a high vessel density. Of patients with recurrent disease, those with high capillary density survived a mean of 45 months vs. 64 months for those with low capillary density[5].

SONOGRAPHIC ASSESSMENT OF VASCULARITY

Color Doppler sonography depicts the relative vascularity within masses by displaying the number and arrangement of vessels that contain blood flow above a certain threshold. This threshold can be lowered, thereby improving blood flow depiction by using amplitude-based rather than frequency-based color Doppler sonography (CDS)[6]. As opposed to frequency CDS (f-CDS), which is proportional to differences in velocities within a vessel, amplitude CDS (a-CDS) correlates with the relative number of blood elements flowing within a vessel (Figure 1).

Other techniques such as contrast infusion coupled with harmonic imaging have greatly enhanced sonographic depiction of vascularity. Some report visualization of vessels as small as 40μm[7]. The flow dynamics within tumors can be assessed by time–activity curves. Tumors typically have longer uptake and 'dwell' times than normal tissues[8].

Methods for quantitation of the blood flow with amplitude CDS have been tested in inoculated tumors and show good correlation ($r = 0.82$) with microvessel density as determined histologically[9] (Figure 2). It may be possible to apply this method to *in vivo* assessment of vessel density, thereby affording an assessment of malignant growth potential (Figures 2, 3, 4 and 5). This type of *in vivo* assessment may be of clinical importance in determining which

masses may require aggressive tumor treatment[10] (Figure 4). Treatment of aggressive tumors may involve the use of antiangiogenesis factors such as angiostatin, which suppresses tumor growth by limiting the formation of tumor vessels.

The role of color Doppler sonography in the assessment of tumor vascularity therefore seems clinically pertinent, justifying expanded research on this topic.

VASCULARITY OF OVARIAN TUMORS

Once an ovarian tumor augments a vascular network, growth and metastasis can occur. The

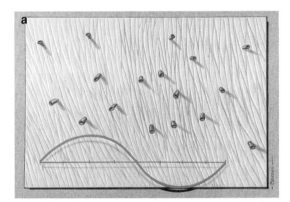

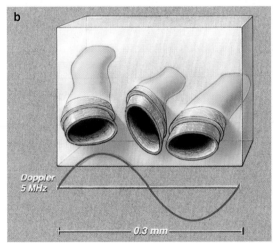

Figure 2 Tumor vascularity. (a) Relative size of tumor vessels compared to wavelength of pulsed Doppler. The flow in several 12–20 μm vessels could construct to produce a Doppler shift. (b) The signals arising from three or more larger (100 μm) tumor vessels may combine to be resolved. (Illustrations by Paul Gross, MS)

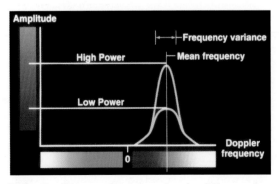

Figure 1 Diagram demonstrating the difference between frequency and amplitude color Doppler sonography (CDS). For a given frequency, better distinction of low and high blood flow can be obtained with amplitude CDS

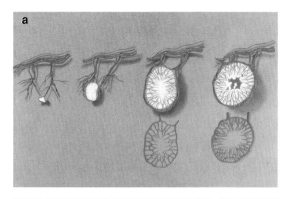
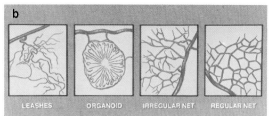
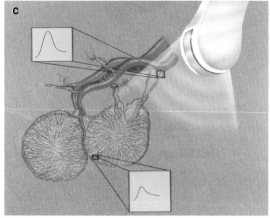
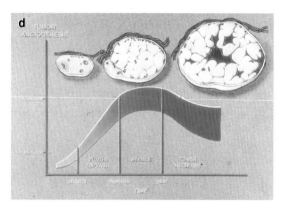

Figure 3 Tumor angiogenesis. (a) Development of tumor neovascularity as the tumor grows to over 2–4 mm. Hemorrhagic necrosis can develop (far right) as the central portion of the tumor outgrows its blood supply. (b) The variety of vessel arrangements in tumors, ranging from a tangle of unorganized vessels to a network of vessels with regular spacing and angulations. Some of these patterns can be recognized on amplitude color Doppler sonography. (c) Diagram showing waveforms from selected vessels in a tumor. The impedance of an intratumoral vessel is lower than that from a 'feeding vessel'. (d) Relative vascularity of ovarian tumors. The tumor is most vascular in the early stages and may become hypovascular with tumor necrosis. (Illustrations by Paul Gross, MS)

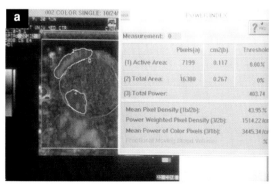
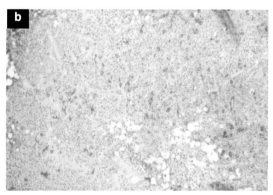

Figure 4 Quantification of vascularity with color Doppler sonography. (a) Composite image and quantification of the vascularity of an implanted tumor. The red line delineates the central portion of the tumor(s); a cluster of vessels in the central portion is shown as 2. A large peripheral vessel is denoted as 1. The power-weighted pixel density ($1514.221/cm^2$) takes into account the number of colorized pixels and weights the flow according to a color scale. (b) Stained specimen, showing an abundance of peripheral vessels and smaller vessels in the center of the tumor

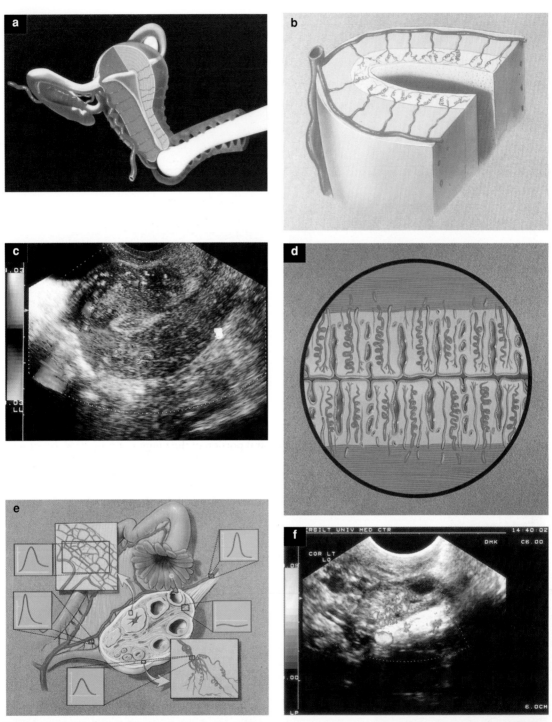

Figure 5 (a) Uterine and ovarian arterial flow. The uterus is supplied by the uterine artery, which is a branch of the hypogastric artery. It courses along the side of the uterus, giving off arcuate branches. The arcuate artery branches into radial arteries and ends as spiral arteries within the endometrium (diagram (b); color Doppler sonography (c)). Within the endometrium, spiral arteries branch into vessels that course within the basalis and functionalis layers (d). The ovarian arterial vessels arise from the main ovarian artery and adnexal branch of the uterine artery (diagram (e); amplitude color Doppler sonography (f)). (Diagrams by Paul Gross, MS)

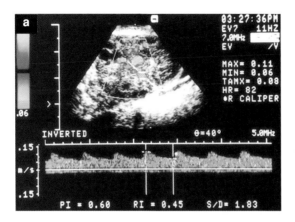

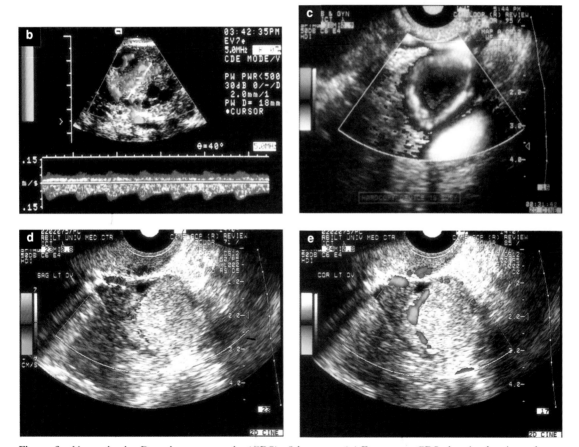

Figure 6 Normal color Doppler sonography (CDS) of the ovary. (a) Frequency CDS, showing low-impedance flow in the wall vessel of the corpus luteum. (b) Amplitude CDS, showing similar low-impedance flow within a corpus luteum. (c) Amplitude CDS, showing circumferential flow (courtesy of Anna Parsons, MD). Frequency CDS (d) and amplitude CDS (e) of solid mass within the left ovary with no central flow. This was a hemorrhagic corpus luteum cyst

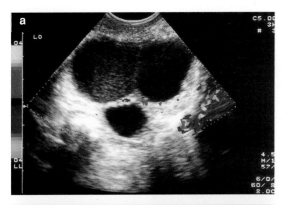

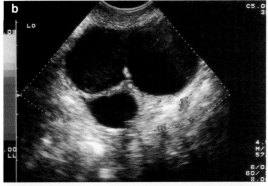

Figure 7 Frequency and amplitude color Doppler sonography (CDS) of a multiloculated hemorrhagic corpus luteum cyst. (a) Frequency CDS of multiloculated mass. Low-level echoes are present within one of the locules. (b) Amplitude CDS of the same multiloculated mass seen in (a). More of the vascularity within the wall of the hemorrhagic locule is apparent

vascularity of rapidly growing tumor is disorganized, with abnormal branching patterns from the host vasculature. Areas of stenoses, microaneurysms and arteriovenous stunts have been indirectly observed on computer-reconstructed microsections[11]. The differences between normal and tumor vascular networks should be a topic of further investigation. This feature may become apparent with the use of contrast agents coupled with harmonic imaging.

CDS findings will depend upon the stage of growth in which the tumor is examined. In the earliest and most rapid stages of development, extensive neovascularity can be observed, whereas as the tumor outgrows its blood supply, it may become relatively hypovascular (Figure 3d).

One must be aware of the variety of waveforms that can be obtained from the ovaries in normally ovulating women (Figure 6). In areas of no follicular development, the intra-ovarian vessels are coiled and demonstrate high impedance, whereas in areas of corpus luteum, low impedance is seen as a reflection of the highly developed network of microvessels within the wall of a functioning corpus luteum (Figure 6b).

Amplitude CDS improves the detection of the microvascularity of ovarian tumors[6] (Figures 7, 8, 9 and 10). Quantification and depiction of the overall blood flow should enhance the ability to distinguish normal from abnormal vessel arrangements with CDS. Pharmacological evaluation of ovarian masses may also be helpful, since tumor vessels should not have the vascular tone of normal vessels.

VASCULARITY OF ENDOMETRIAL TUMORS

The endometrium in women of childbearing age contains a highly vascular network, particularly in the secretory phase (Figure 5). With amplitude CDS, the microscopic spiral arteries that lie between the glandular elements of the secretory-phase endometrium can be seen. With menses, the hypovascular endometrium is shed. Similarly, in postmenopausal women, the endometrium should appear relatively hypovascular. With hyperplasia, or cancer, the endometrium becomes vascular. Instead of spontaneously regressing, the endometrial microvascularity in hyperplasia and cancer enlarges and becomes more intertwined. There have been ultrastructural observations that the endometrial microvascularity in hyperplasia consists of extensive proliferation of immature capillaries that are disorganzied when compared to those of the normal endometrium[12].

In order to understand the CDS findings that are observed, one should be aware of the microscopic changes in the uterine and endometrial vasculature that occur during the menstrual cycle[13]. At the time of menstruation, the spiral arteries constrict, as a response to decreasing

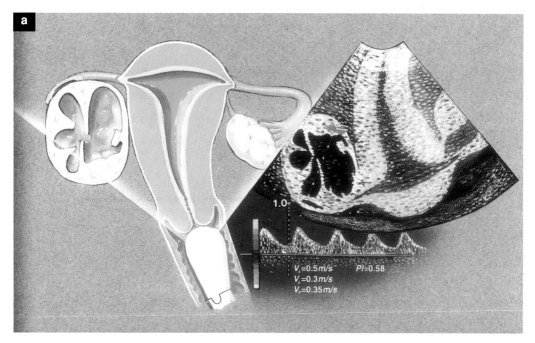

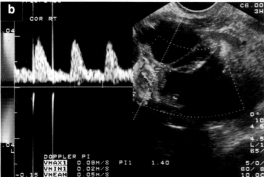

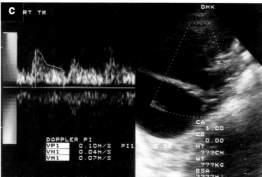

Figure 8 (a) Diagram of transvaginal color Doppler sonography of a multiseptated ovarian mass. The triplex image consists of a real-time transvaginal image combined with duplex Doppler and waveform (Diagram by Paul Gross, MS). (b) Benign cystadenoma with high impedance (PI = 1.4). (c) Cystadenocarcinoma with low impedance (PI = 0.86)

estrogen and progesterone levels. This produces local hypoxia, ischemia and eventually cell death within the stratum functionalis. The distal portion of the arteriolar system, as well as the capillary and venous beds, are then shed with the functionalis. The local arteries, which are relatively insensitive to decreasing estrogen and progesterone levels, are relatively unaffected and serve to maintain the integrity of the stratum basalis throughout the menstrual cycle. As the endometrium thickens three- to five-fold

during the next menstrual cycle, the remnants of the spiral arteries in the basalis must undergo substantial growth and give rise to a completely new capillary bed in order to maintain the integrity of the rapidly growing stroma. This process is initiated by the growth of new capillaries from the existing vasculature in the basalis. These capillaries eventually differentiate into arteries and arterioles as the elastic and vascular smooth muscle component develops around the new capillaries.

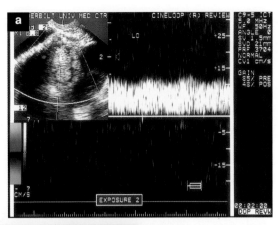

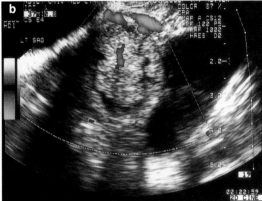

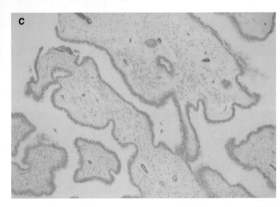

Figure 9 Color Doppler sonography (CDS) of cystic masses with papillary excrescence. (a) Frequency CDS of enlarged left ovary with highly vascular solid area within papillary excrescence of an ovarian papillary cancer. (b) Magnified amplitude CDS of the ovarian mass in (a), showing vessel within papillary excrescence. (c) Low-power photomicrograph, showing vessels within tumor papilla

Although incompletely understood, the angiogenesis that occurs with endometrial hyperplasia and carcinoma is probably initiated by elaboration of growth factors and/or reduced production of an inhibitory regulator. Microscopically, the tumor vessels have incomplete basement membranes and are leaky. These features may become increasingly apparent on CDS with the use of contrast and possibly pharmacological enhancement.

More extensive experience is required for accurate assessment of the specificity and sensitivity of CDS for the detection of endometrial tumors. However, our initial experience has shown that CDS findings seem to correspond with the observation of increased vascularity of these tumors as seen on histology. Focal areas of increased vascularity may be observed in the vascular pedicle of polyps (Figure 11). Increased vascularity may also be the result of inflammation with vasodilatation as the basic mechanism for this increase in flow.

CONCLUSION

CDS depiction of tumor angiogenesis has many clinical implications, including early detection of ovarian and endometrial cancers. Improved detection and quantification of flow with CDS can hopefully contribute to a reduction in morbidity and mortality from these two cancers.

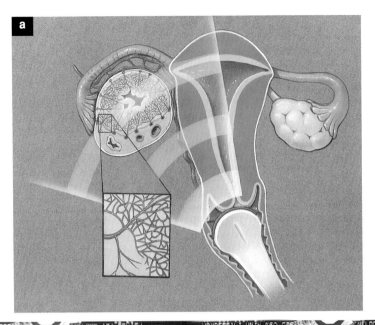

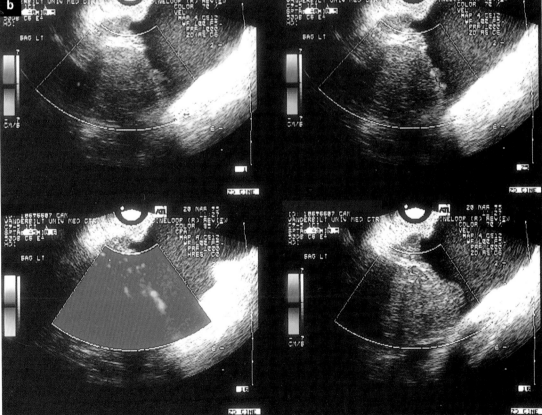

Figure 10 (a) Drawing, showing tumor vascularity in a solid ovarian cancer. The tumor vessels branch in a disorganized fashion (Drawing by Paul Gross, MS). (b) Composite image, showing vascularity within a solid adnexal mass. Note the disorganized cluster of vessels within the mass, best depicted by amplitude color Doppler sonography (CDS) in the lower left image. *Continued on p. 110*

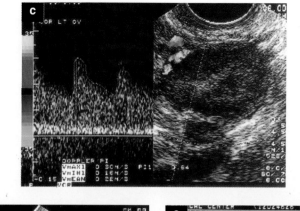

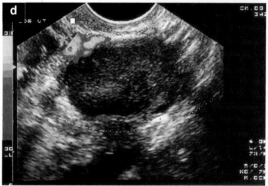
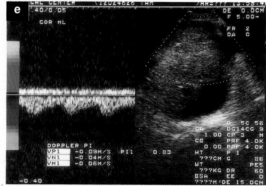

Figure 10 *continued* (c) Frequency CDS of a solid mass with low-impedance flow. (d) Amplitude CDS of same mass shown in (c), depicting peripheral vessels within this metastatic lesion to the ovary. (e) Frequency CDS of an adnexal mass seen in a patient during the first trimester of pregnancy. There was low-impedance flow in the solid area of this ovarian carcinoma

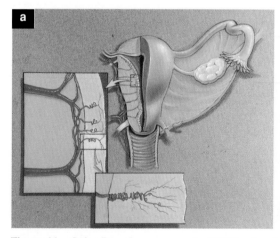
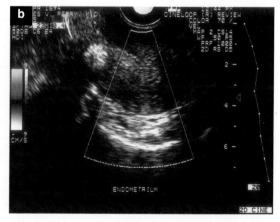

Figure 11 Color Doppler sonography (CDS) of endometrial disorders. (a) Diagram, showing endometrial arterial supply. The radial arteries arise from the arcuate arteries, which are branches of the uterine arteries, which course along the uterine corpus. The spiral arteries are branches of the radial arteries. *Continued*

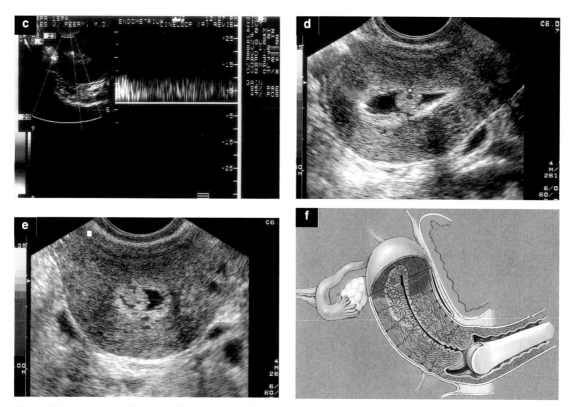

Figure 11 *continued* (b and c) Transvaginal CDS of endometrial hyperplasia, showing venous flow within a thickened endometrium (courtesy of C. Peery, MD). CDS, showing vascularity within the pedicle of an endometrial polyp as imaged in long (d) and short (e) axes during sonohysterography. (f) Drawing of the tumor vascularity within an endometrial cancer (Drawing by Paul Gross, MS)

References

1. Kurjak, A., Shalan, H., Kupesic, S. *et al.* (1994). An attempt to screen asymptomatic women for ovarian and endometrial cancer with transvaginal color and pulsed Doppler sonography. *J. Ultrasound Med.*, **13**, 295–301

2. Fleischer, A., Cullinan, J., Peery, C. and Jones, H. (1996). Early detection of ovarian carcinoma with transvaginal color Doppler ultrasonography. *Am. J. Obstet. Gynecol.*, **174**, 101–6

3. Weidner, N. (1995). Intratumor microvessel density as a prognostic factor in cancer. *Am. J. Pathol.*, **147**, 9–19

4. Hollingsworth, H., Kohn, E., Steinberg, S., Rothenberg, M. L. and Merino, M. J. (1995). Tumor angiogenesis in advanced stage ovarian carcinoma. *Am. J. Pathol.*, **147**, 33–41

5. Kirschner, C. V., Alanis-Amezcua, J. M., Martin, V. G., Luna, N., Morgan, E., Yang, J. J. and Yordan, E. L. (1996). Angiogenesis factor in endometrial carcinoma: a new prognostic indicator? *Am. J. Obstet. Gynecol.*, **174**, 1879–84

6. Fleischer, A., Johnson, J. and Tait, D. (1996). Amplitude and frequency based transvaginal color Doppler sonography of ovarian masses: correlation with microvascularity. *Ultrasound Int.*, **3**, 118–21

7. Burns, P. (1995). Harmonic imaging adds to ultrasound capabilities. *Diagn. Imaging* (Suppl.), AU7–9

8. Cosgrove, D. (1997). Evaluation of tumors using echo enhancing agents. In Goldberg, B. (ed.) *Ultrasound Contrast Agents*, pp. 159–69. (London: Martin Dunitz)

9. Meyerowitz, C. B., Fleischer, A. C., Pickens, D. R., Thurman, G. B., Borowsky, A. D., Thirsk, G. and Hellerqvist, C. G. (1996). Quantification

of tumor vascularity and flow with amplitude color Doppler sonography in an experimental model: preliminary results. *J. Ultrasound Med.*, **15**, 827–33

10. Folkman, J. (1995). Clinical applications of research on angiogenesis. *N. Engl. J. Med.*, **333**, 1757–63

11. Schoenfeld, A., Levavi, H., Tepper, R., Breslavski, D., Amir, R. and Ovadia, J. (1994). Assessment of tumor-induced angiogenesis by three-dimensional display: confusing Doppler signals in ovarian cancer screening? *Ultrasound Obstet. Gynecol.*, **4**, 516–18

12. Horbelt, D., Roberts, D., Parmley, T. and Walker, N. (1996). Ultrastructure of the microvasculature in human endometrial hyperplasia. *Am. J. Obstet. Gynecol.*, **174**, 174–83

13. Torry, R. and Rongish, B. J. (1992). Angiogenesis in the uterus: potential regulation and relation to tumor angiogenesis. Review. *Am. J. Reprod. Immun.*, **27**, 171–9

Myometrial invasion of endometrial carcinoma evaluated by amplitude color Doppler sonohysterography

10

S. Fujiwaki and B. Ishizuka

There have been attempts to utilize endovaginal sonography for the evaluation of myometrial invasion of endometrial carcinoma[1]. However, with conventional endovaginal sonography, it is often difficult to clearly visualize the extent of the carcinoma growth into the myometrium (Figure 1). We have therefore examined the diagnostic value of sonohysterography[2–4] with amplitude color Doppler sonography (CDS) in determining the degree of myometrial invasion.

Sonohysterography was performed by GE, LOGIQ 500 MD with amplitude CDS and 6.5-MHz endovaginal probe. A flexible Foley 8.0 French balloon catheter was introduced into the cervical canal, and the endometrial cavity was dilated with 10% glucose solution by drip infusion from about 30 cm above the level of the uterine cavity to prevent the solution from overflowing into the peritoneal cavity[5]. A balloon was fixed in the cervical canal so that it would not damage the endometrium and obstruct the sonographic view of the lower portion of the uterine cavity.

With fluid collection in the uterine cavity, the localization of the portion of the tumor protruding into the endometrial cavity becomes much easier (Figure 2). When the carcinoma has spread over the endometrial surface, localization of the tumor by sonohysterography becomes more difficult. In such cases, detection of increased vascularity from the normal endometrium to the endometrial cancer by amplitude CDS can facilitate the delineation of the cancer invasion.

Carcinoma invasion into the endometrium can be estimated by the increased vascularity surrounding the carcinoma tissue; however, the extent of the invasion is often overestimated

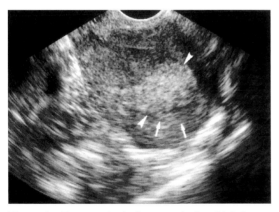

Figure 1 Transvaginal ultrasound: the thick hyperechoic endometrium (arrowheads) is noted. The halo (arrows) cannot be clearly visualized in the anterior superior portion of the uterus

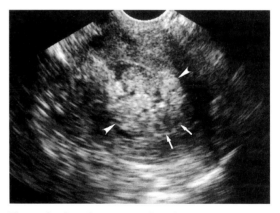

Figure 2 Sonohysterography: the uterine cavity is occupied by irregular and thick hyperechoic areas (arrowheads). In the uterine fundus, the margin of the hyperechoic area and myometrium is obscure, suggesting myometrial invasion (arrows)

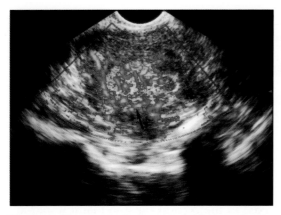

Figure 3 Transvaginal ultrasound with amplitude CDS: the color flow map is noted (arrow) from myometrium to thick hyperechoic endometrium

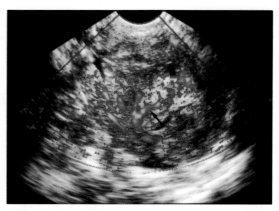

Figure 4 Sonohysterography with amplitude CDS: the color flow map is noted (arrow) from myometrium to thick hyperechoic endometrium, which is suggested to be myometrial invasion

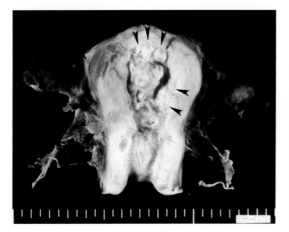

Figure 5 Macroscopic findings: the tumor (arrowheads) invaded to one-third of the myometrium in the uterine fundus

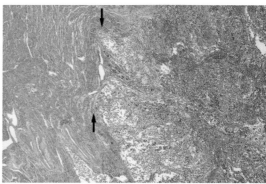

Figure 6 Histological findings (hematoxylin–eosin): the cancer (arrows) invaded to one-third of the uterine myometrium

when it is evaluated only with amplitude CDS. With sonohysterography, the myometrial invasion is demonstrated by the disruption of the halo and a change in the echogenicity of the myometrium. In combination with sonohystero-graphy, amplitude CDS can delineate nutrient vessels supplying the carcinoma tissue more clearly; this leads to more precise delineation of the extent of the invasion (Figures 3, 4, 5 and 6).

References

1. Fleischer, A. C., Dudley, B. S. and Entman, S. S. (1987). Myometrial invasion by endometrial cancer: sonographic assessment. *Radiology*, **162**, 307–10

2. Deichert, U., van de Sandt, M., Lauth, G. and Daume, E. (1988). Transvaginal contrast hysterosonography. A new diagnostic procedure for the differentiation of intrauterine and myometrial findings. *Geburtshilfe Frauenheikd*, **48**, 835–44

3. Parsons, A. K. and Lense, J. J. (1993). Sonohysterography for endometrial abnormalities: preliminary results. *J. Clin. Ultrasound*, **21**, 97–105
4. Fujiwaki, S., Saito, J., Horokoshi, H., Ishizuka, B., Amemiya, A. and Sakuyama, K. (1995). Diagnosis of intrauterine disorders by sonohysterography. *Acta Obstet. Gynaecol. Jpn.*, **47**, 437–40

5. Sagawa, T., Yamada, H., Sakuragi, N. and Fujimoto, S. (1994). A comparison between the preoperative and operative findings of peritoneal cytology in patients with endometrial cancer. *Asia-Oceania J. Obstet. Gynecol.*, **20**, 39–47

Doppler assessment of uterine myomas

11

H. Yun, A. Sosic and F. A. Chervenak

INTRODUCTION

Uterine myomas are the most common neoplasms of the female pelvis and occur in 20–25% of women of reproductive age[1]. Approximately 30% of all hysterectomies and an undetermined number of major and minor conservative surgical procedures are performed for myomas.

Uterine myomas occur and grow in women during the reproductive years and decrease in size after menopause or after oophorectomy. Recent trials of gonadotropin releasing hormone (GnRH) agonists, documenting significant reduction in tumor size by the production of a hypogonadal state, have provided additional evidence of the hormone sensitivity of myomas.

The diagnosis can be established with very high confidence on the basis of bimanual examination alone, which usually reveals an enlarged, firm, non-tender and irregularly contoured uterus. Sometimes, an alternative pathology, including benign and malignant ovarian neoplasm, endometriosis, adenomyosis, or inflammatory masses, may be found in patients surgically treated for presumed myomas. Differentiation from ovarian tumors is essential and becomes extremely difficult when the pelvic mass is large and totally fills the pelvis.

Diagnostic accuracy has improved since the advent of modern imaging technologies. Transabdominal and transvaginal ultrasound are the standard imaging modalities for the detection of myomas. Transvaginal ultrasound is more sensitive in obese patients, as well as in patients with small myomas or a retroverted uterus. Large uteri or masses lie outside the focal zone of the endovaginal transducer and are best observed via the transabdominal approach.

Recently, transvaginal fluid-enhanced ultrasound (sonohysterography) has been suggested as a very useful modality for the evaluation of submucous myomas[2]. In 1985, Taylor and co-workers[3] used transabdominal pulsed Doppler ultrasound to measure blood flow indices in the uterine and ovarian arteries. Color Doppler ultrasound was also developed in the mid-1980s, initially as a technique for cardiac investigation[4]. A few years later, its use was expanded to other areas of the human circulation. In 1987, Kurjak and co-workers[5] introduced transvaginal color Doppler ultrasound for the assessment of the pelvic circulation. The development of endovaginal probes, which involve the use of higher-frequency ultrasound for imaging and pulsed Doppler, has facilitated studies of angiogenesis within pelvic tumors. The first studies on the use of color Doppler ultrasound to differentiate between benign and malignant pelvic tumors have revealed interesting results. Malignant pelvic tumors were characterized by areas of angiogenesis that produced high-velocity, low-resistance blood flow, whereas most benign tumors were not[6,7]. Subsequently, larger studies confirmed that some benign tumors have the same features as malignant tumors when imaged by color Doppler ultrasound[8]. In some cases, this was explained by the presence of inflammation in a benign tumor. However, there were other benign tumors that were not associated with inflammation that possessed these features. The histopathological evaluation of blood vessels was not used to explain these various vascular patterns. It is still not clear whether persistent vasodilation of host vessels may produce the typical high-velocity, low-resistance waveforms usually associated with angiogenesis. Transvaginal color Doppler ultrasound is increasing in use in patients with uterine disorders. The characterization of endometrial pathology and the evaluation of hormone and drug effects on the uterus are at present its main applications in these patients.

BIOLOGY OF UTERINE MYOMAS

Uterine myomas are benign neoplasms that arise from a single progenitor cell[9]. Multiple myomas within the same uterus are not clonally related; each myoma arises independently. Different rates of growth can reflect the different cytogenetic abnormalities present in individual tumors[10]. A variety of substances stimulate the growth of uterine myomas, including insulin-like growth factors I and II[11], epidermal growth factor[12], growth hormone[13], estrogen[14] and progestagens[14]. The environment within the myoma is hyperestrogenic. Endometrial hyperplasia is frequently observed at the margins of a submucous myoma[15]. The smooth muscle cells of uterine myomas produce prostaglandins as well as large amounts of prostacyclin[16]. These agents alter uterine vascular tone and uterine contractility and may be responsible for uterine dysfunctional activity. Myomas contain elevated levels of prolactin, which is identical to pituitary and decidual prolactin. The symptomatic hyperprolactinemia caused by this prolactin is rare and is unresponsive to bromocriptin[17]. Myomas may produce erythropoietin, resulting in an elevation of the hematocrit and polycytemia[18].

CLASSIFICATION

Myomas are usually multiple benign tumors of various sizes, surrounded by a pseudocapsule of compressed muscle fibers. A single nodule is found in only 2% of patients[19]. Myomas usually develop in the uterine corpus and fundus; only 3% are of cervical origin[19]. They are classified according to their position in the uterus. The most common are intramural, located within the uterine wall. Submucous myomas are under the endometrium and protrude into the endometrial cavity. Subserous myomas are located beneath the uterine serosa and produce asymmetric uterine irregularity. These tumors may occasionally be intraligamentous, growing from the uterus into the broad ligament. Both submucous and subserous myomas may become pedunculated and undergo torsion, with subsequent degeneration and potential infection. Pedunculated subserous tumors that outgrow their uterine blood supply and obtain a secondary blood supply from another organ, such as omentum, are termed parasitic myomas.

CLINICAL ASPECTS

The majority of myomas are asymptomatic. The most common symptom associated with myomas is abnormal bleeding, which typically presents as menorrhagia. The mechanism of the myoma-associated bleeding is unknown. Alterations in the endometrial microvasculature, such as venular ectasia or dilatation, have been observed in these patients[1].

Chronic pelvic pain is rarely caused by myomas. Acute pelvic pain, associated with low-grade fever and localized uterine tenderness, may be observed either with carneous degeneration or, more rarely, with torsion of pedunculated tumors.

A large myomatous uterus may produce urinary frequency and hydronephrosis, may interfere with bowel movements, or may produce a heavy feeling or general discomfort in the pelvis. These symptoms are common indications for surgical treatment.

A variety of reproductive disorders, including infertility, habitual abortion and preterm labor, have been attributed to uterine myomas. Most studies that made this association were not controlled for the patient's age, position and size of the myomas or other factors affecting fertility and pregnancy outcome. Uterine myomas that interfere neither with tubal structure nor the endometrium and its underlying myometrial architecture are unlikely to result in infertility.

SONOGRAPHIC FEATURES

Sonographically, myomas are hypoechoic, isoechoic or hyperechoic, compared to normal myometrium. The echogenicity depends on the ratio of connective tissue to muscle fibers. With a more fibrous component, there is increased echogenicity of the nodule. The echogenicity also depends on the presence and type of degeneration and vascular supply. Alteration in the blood supply to uterine myomas, which can occur with changes in a woman's hormonal status, can produce a variety of degenerative changes. The most common is hyaline degeneration and appears as anechoic areas within a myoma. Calcification is more common in postmenopausal women. It can be diffuse, localized, or present only on the surface of the tumors. It can be recognized as clusters of high-level echoes that produce distal acoustic shadowing. Cystic degeneration produces anechoic areas within a myoma as well as posterior wall enhancement, differentiating it from hyaline degeneration. Uterine myomas occasionally become infected. On rare occasions, the infection may even produce abscesses within the tumor (pyomyoma).

VASCULAR ANATOMY OF THE UTERUS

The uterus derives its blood supply from the uterine artery, a direct branch of the hypogastric artery. The main uterine artery courses medially towards the cervicocorporeal junction, where it bifurcates into an ascending and descending branch. The ascending branch passes within the broad ligament along the lateral wall of the uterus towards the uterotubal junction. The ascending branch is a very tortuous vessel in the non-gravid uterus. The arcuate arteries lie at the level of the junction between the outer and middle thirds of the myometrium and run circumferentially around the uterine wall. The arcuate arteries give off branches, the radial arteries, that course in a configuration resembling the spokes of a wheel towards the endometrium. The branches of radial vessels are of two types: (1) straight arteries, which supply the stratum basalis; and (2) spiral arteries, highly tortuous vessels that supply the stratum spongiosum and stratum compactum[20]. Transvaginal color Doppler ultrasound easily depicts the main uterine and arcuate vessels in almost all patients. More distal branches cannot be seen in all patients. Visualization of these vessels is improved by the administration of substances that dilate them.

UTERINE PERFUSION

The development of endovaginal probes, which involve the use of higher-frequency ultrasound for imaging and pulsed Doppler, have facilitated studies of blood flow in uterine arteries. Transvaginal color Doppler can be used to measure impedance to blood flow in the uterine arteries reproducibly, and the characteristic flow velocity waveforms obtained from these vessels have been described[21]. In the last decade, the Doppler technique has been extensively used for the study of uterine perfusion in many physiological and pathological conditions. These conditions include: spontaneous and artificial menstrual cycles, the uterine vasculature under the effects of various drugs, spontaneous and artificially induced menopause, hormone replacement therapy, characterization of uterine tumors and medical treatment of uterine myomas.

During the normal menstrual cycle, the lowest impedance to uterine blood flow occurs at the start of rapid follicular growth 6 days before the luteinizing hormone (LH) peak and subsequently during peak luteal function, around the presumed time when implantation might occur. The peak impedance to uterine blood flow is around the time of menses and this high impedance persists during the development of a preovulatory follicle[21]. It has been shown that measurement of the mean uterine arterial pulsatility index (PI) shortly before embryo transfer (ET) is a useful method of assessing uterine receptivity during the treatment of infertility by *in vitro* fertilization (IVF) and ET[22]. During spontaneously induced menopause there is a decrease in uterine perfusion with a progressive increase of the PI with duration of menopause[23]. The PI in uterine arteries also increases in patients with artificially induced menopause[23]. When used for hormone replacement therapy, estrogen rapidly reduces the impedance to blood flow in the uterine artery, whereas the addition of progestagens partially reverses this drop in impedance[24,25]. Both benign and malignant tumors also influence uterine perfusion by increasing uterine artery blood flow and lowering resistance to blood flow[26].

THE CHARACTERIZATION OF UTERINE TUMORS

Uterine arteries are amenable to study by Doppler ultrasound in all patients, whereas the blood vessels within myomas are not. This was obvious in the first published reports[5,6], when a significant number of studied myomas were found to be 'avascular'. The reasons for this lie in technical limitations (the myoma is not in the focal range of the transducer) as well as the sensitivity of the equipment used. In our experience, combined use of both transabdominal and transvaginal approaches results in the finding of a smaller number of 'avascular' myomas.

Several investigators used transvaginal color Doppler to discriminate benign from malignant uterine tumors. Kurjak and Zalud[27] studied a group of 308 patients with uterine tumors. The blood flow was visualized in 58% of myomas, with mean resistance index (RI) equal to 0.58. They concluded that vascularization of uterine myomas is supported by normal existing vessels. When color flow was present, waveform analysis indicated blood velocities similar to the normal myometrial perfusion originating from terminal branches of the uterine artery. Their ability to demonstrate tumor vessels was dependent on the tumor size and position, as well as the extent of secondary degenerative changes. In three cases of uterine sarcoma, the visualization of blood flow was 100% and the mean RI was 0.31. Subsequently, the significance of the location of blood vessels within tumor was described. The neovascularization within tumor tissue is of the peripheral and/or central vessel type. A lower impedance in central vessels than in peripheral

vessels was observed in both benign and malignant tumors[28,29].

Not all investigators have agreed that color Doppler ultrasound can be used clinically to differentiate benign from malignant uterine tumors. In one study[30] that included 122 patients with suspected uterine pathology, there was no difference between the benign and malignant groups for the systolic, diastolic and mean velocities or for the calculated PI and RI in either uterine or tumor vessels. Using a cut-off level of 1.0 for the PI, the sensitivity, specificity, positive predictive value and negative predictive value were 34%, 73%, 50% and 58%, respectively. The authors concluded that color Doppler is generally not helpful in distinguishing benign from malignant uterine tumors. In the largest published study that used transvaginal color Doppler to differentiate benign from malignant uterine tumors, Kurjak and colleagues[31] examined a group of 2010 women 1 day before planned hysterectomy. The findings in 10 cases of uterine sarcoma were compared to those in 1850 myoma uteri. All cases of uterine sarcoma (100%) revealed abnormal tumor blood flow. The mean RI of these vessels was 0.37 (range 0.32–0.42). Using a cut-off point of 0.40 for the RI, the authors were able to distinguish between benign and malignant myometrial tumors with a sensitivity of 90.9%, specificity of 99.8%, positive predictive value of 71% and negative predictive value of 99.96%.

Other investigators have concluded that myomas substantially affect blood flow velocity in the uterine arteries and that a low PI in tumor vessels is not an unusual finding and does not necessarily indicate malignancy[32].

Sosic and co-workers[33] used color Doppler ultrasound to study the vascularity of uterine myomas in a group of 195 patients. A total number of 405 myomas, 316 in premenopausal and 89 in postmenopausal patients, were studied by this technique. The mean RI in the myoma vessels was significantly lower in the premenopausal group (RI = 0.64) than in the postmenopausal group (RI = 0.70). The size of the myoma was the most important single factor in determining both the blood flow visualization rate and the RI (Table 1). With the increase in

Table 1 Blood flow visualization rate (BFVR) and resistance index (RI) as a function of the menopausal status of the patient and the size of the myoma. From reference 33, with permission

Size of myoma (mm)	Premenopausal			Postmenopausal		
	Myomas (n)	BFVR (%)	RI	Myomas (n)	BFVR (%)	RI
< 20	117	36	0.66 ± 0.11	29	14	0.77 ± 0.16
20–40	111	59	0.66 ± 0.10	41	54	0.70 ± 0.08
> 40	88	77	0.60 ± 0.13	19	95	0.68 ± 0.14
Total	316	55	0.64 ± 0.12	89	49	0.70 ± 0.11

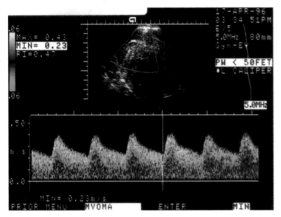

Figure 1 Large myomas are frequently characterized by a high-velocity, low impedance blood flow pattern (RI = 0.47, V_{max} = 43 cm/s)

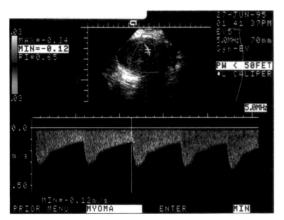

Figure 2 This high-velocity (V_{max} = 34 cm/s), high-impedance (RI = 0.65) flow is, in our experience, the most frequent color Doppler finding associated with uterine myomas

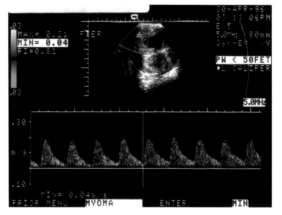

Figure 3 GnRH agonist treatment: cystic degeneration within the myoma secondary to the diminished blood supply. After completion of treatment, a high-impedance flow is typically seen in these patients. RI = 0.81

Table 2 Distribution of resistance index (RI) values in the study group. From reference 33, with permission

RI	Myoma			
	Premenopausal		Postmenopausal	
≤ 0.40	4	(1%)	0	(0%)
0.41–0.50	26	(8%)	4	(4%)
0.51–0.60	39	(12%)	3	(3%)
> 0.60	106	(34%)	37	(42%)
No flow	141	(45%)	45	(51%)
Total	316	(100%)	89	(100%)

size, a decrease in RI was seen only in subserous and submucous locations (Figure 1). The lowest RI values were noted in submucous and subserous myomas larger than 40 mm. In general, the majority of myomas exhibited high resistance to blood flow (Figure 2), characterized either by non-visualization of flow or by an RI of > 0.60 (Table 2). The duration of menopause and the phase of the cycle in the menstruating women did not significantly affect the measured

Doppler parameters, suggesting that the mechanisms of regulation of blood flow within myomas may not be the same as those in the uterine arteries.

It appears that the size of the myoma is an important factor in determining both visualization of flow and RI. The pressure from the surrounding healthy myometrium on the tumor may be one of the reasons for an increased impedance to flow in intramural myomas. Also, differing physiology of the surrounding tissue (i.e. myometrium vs. endometrium vs. peritoneum) and the proximity to the large branches of the uterine artery may have had an effect on the studied Doppler parameters.

Leiomyosarcoma is a *de novo* neoplasm which does not represent a degenerative change arising in a pre-existing benign myoma. Women with myomas do not appear to be at a higher risk for leiomyosarcoma. The incidence of sarcoma among patients with presumed myomas is about 1 : 500[34]. This event is so uncommon that, until now, its possibility has not influenced the clinical management of a patient with myomas. The presenting symptoms of both tumor types are the same and include uterine bleeding, pelvic pain and/or pelvic mass. Uterine sarcoma should be considered in all postmenopausal patients who have these symptoms and a rapidly enlarging uterine mass. In one study[35], leiomyosarcoma was the largest uterine mass in more than 50% of patients having this disease and in the other 30% it was the only uterine mass present. Preoperative diagnosis of leiomyosarcoma was difficult and it was usually not established until the surgical specimen was evaluated histologically. The introduction of transvaginal ultrasound, equipped with a high-resolution transducer, is promising in terms of evaluating more detailed sonomorphological patterns of uterine tumors. Attention should be directed to the dominant myoma during conservative management. It has been shown previously that leiomyosarcomas, as a result of increased neovascularization, have lower impedance to blood flow compared with benign myomas. It was demonstrated that, by using a cut-off level of 0.40 for the RI, it is possible to achieve a high sensitivity and specificity in discriminating malignant from benign uterine tumors. In one study[31], five asymptomatic myomas had an RI of ≤ 0.40, indicating possible limitations of a lower RI to discriminate between uterine myoma and a true sarcoma. In the same paper, Kurjak and co-workers[31] suggested a more comprehensive evaluation of uterine tumors that should include assessments of sonomorphology, vascular anatomy and the Doppler waveform. We believe that such an approach will improve the effectiveness of this technique.

MEDICAL THERAPY OF UTERINE MYOMAS

Probably one of the most useful applications of color Doppler ultrasound in patients with uterine disorders is in the assessment of uterine perfusion before and after medical treatment of uterine myomas. In 1983, Filicori and associates[36] reported that the administration of a GnRH agonist reduced the size of uterine myomas. For the first time, the advent of these drugs has allowed effective medical therapy for uterine myomas. The average shrinkage of myomas is more than 50%, but the range for individual tumors varies from no change to more than 90%. Maximum tumor shrinkage occurs by 8 to 12 weeks of therapy[37,38]. Using color Doppler ultrasound, several authors[39,40] were able to demonstrate an increase in impedance to blood flow and a decrease in blood flow velocity in both uterine and tumor blood vessels (Figure 3). The individual differences in response to these drugs are possibly caused by the differences in size and location of the myoma, as well as differences in vascularity and impedance to blood flow within these tumors. Further studies should evaluate whether careful sonographic assessment of these parameters may predict the response to treatment and its optimal duration. Larger submucous and subserous myomas may represent especially good targets for treatment with these drugs. This could have positive effects on their subsequent surgical removal.

References

1. American College of Obstetricians and Gynecologists (1994). *Uterine Leiomyomata. ACOG Technical Bulletin 192.* (Washington, DC: ACOG)

2. Fukuda, M., Shimizu, T., Fukuda, K., Yomura, W. and Shimizu, S. (1993). Transvaginal hysterosonography for differential diagnosis between submucous and intramural myoma. *Gynecol. Obstet. Invest.*, **35**, 236–9

3. Taylor, K. J., Burns, P. N., Wells, P. N., Conway, D. I. and Hull, M. G. (1985). Ultrasound Doppler flow studies of the ovarian and uterine arteries. *Br. J. Obstet. Gynaecol.*, **92**, 240–6

4. Omoto, R. (1984). *Color Atlas of Two-dimensional Doppler Echocardiography.* (Tokyo: Shirdan-To-Chiryo)

5. Kurjak, A., Zalud, I., Jurkovic, D., Alfirevic, D. and Miljan, M. (1989). Transvaginal color Doppler for the assessment of pelvic circulation. *Acta Obstet. Gynecol. Scand.*, **68**, 131–5

6. Kurjak, A., Jurkovic, D., Alfirevic, D. and Zalud, I. (1990). Transvaginal color Doppler imaging. *J. Clin. Ultrasound*, **18**, 227–31

7. Hata, T., Hata, K., Senoch, D., Makihara, K., Aoki, S., Takamiya, O., Kitao, M. and Umaki, K. (1990). Transvaginal Doppler flow mapping. *Gynecol. Obstet. Invest.*, **27**, 217–18

8. Kurjak, A., Shalan, H., Kupesic, S., Predanic, M., Zalud, I., Breyer, B. and Jukic, S. (1993). Transvaginal color Doppler sonography in the assessment of pelvic tumor vascularity. *Ultrasound Obstet. Gynecol.*, **3**, 1–15

9. Townsend, D. E., Sparkes, R. S., Baluda, M. C. and McClelland, G. (1970). Unicellular histogenesis of uterine leiomyomas as determined by electrophoresis of glucose-6-phosphate dehydrogenase. *Am. J. Obstet. Gynecol.*, **107**, 1168–73

10. Nilbert, M. and Heim, S. (1990). Uterine leiomyoma cytogenetics. *Genes Chromosom. Cancer*, **2**, 3–13

11. Chandrasekhar, Y., Heiner, J., Osuampke, C. and Nagamani, M. (1992). Insulin-like growth factor I and II binding in human myometrium and leiomyomas. *Am. J. Obstet. Gynecol.*, **166**, 64–9

12. Fayed, Y. M., Tsibris, J. C. M. and Langenberg, P. Q. (1989). Human uterine leiomyoma cells: binding and growth response to epidermal growth factor, platelet-derived growth factor, and insulin. *Lab. Invest.*, **60**, 30–7

13. Spellacy, W. M., LeMaire, W. J. and Buhl, W. C. (1972). Plasma growth hormone and estradiol levels in women with uterine myomas. *Obstet. Gynecol.*, **40**, 829

14. Soules, M. R. and McCarty, K. S. Jr (1982). Leiomyomas: steroid receptor content. Variation within normal menstrual cycles. *Am. J. Obstet. Gynecol.*, **143**, 6–11

15. Deligdish, L. and Loewenthal, M. (1970). Endometrial changes associated with myomata of the uterus. *J. Clin. Pathol.*, **23**, 676

16. Bamford, D. S., Jorgee, M. and Williams, K. L. (1980). Prostacyclin formation by the pregnant human myometrium. *Br. J. Obstet. Gynaecol.*, **87**, 215–18

17. Kenigsberg, D., Chapitis, J., Zuna, R. and Riddick, D. (1987). Hyperprolactinemia arising from a uterine tumor (abstr.). *Soc. Gynecol. Invest.*, **34**, 157

18. Weiss, D. B., Aldor, A. and Aboulafia, Y. (1975). Erythrocytosis due to erythropoietin-producing uterine fibromyoma. *Am. J. Obstet. Gynecol.*, **122**, 358–60

19. Sanders, R. C. and James, A. E. (1985). *Principles and Practice of Ultrasonography in Obstetrics and Gynecology*, 3rd edn., pp. 540–2. (Norfolk, Connecticut: Appleton Centuary Croft)

20. Burton, G. J. (1995). Vascular anatomy of the pelvis. In Bourne, T. H., Jauniaux, E. and Jurkovic, D. (eds.) *Transvaginal Colour Doppler*, pp. 20–70. (Berlin, Heidelberg: Springer-Verlag)

21. Steer, C. W., Campbell, S., Pampligione, J., Kingsland, C. R., Mason, B. A. and Collins, W. P. (1990). Transvaginal colour flow imaging of the uterine arteries during the ovarian and menstrual cycle. *Hum. Reprod.*, **5**, 391–5

22. Steer, C. V., Campbell, S., Tan, S. L., Crayford, T., Mills, C., Mason, B. A. and Collins, W. P. (1992). The use of transvaginal color flow imaging after *in vitro* fertilization to identify optimum uterine conditions before embryo transfer. *Fertil. Steril.*, **57**, 372–6

23. Luzi, G., Coata, G., Cucchia, C., Cosmi, E. V. and Di Renzo, G. C. (1993). Doppler studies of uterine arteries in spontaneous and artificially induced menopausal women. *Ultrasound Obstet. Gynecol.*, **3**, 354–6

24. Bourne, T. H., Hillard, T., Whitehead, M. I., Crook, D. and Campbell, S. (1990). Evidence for a rapid effect of oestrogens on the arterial status of postmenopausal women. *Lancet*, **335**, 1470–1

25. Hillard, T. C., Bourne, T. H., Crayford, T., Collins, W. P., Campbell, S. and Whitehead, M. I. (1993). Differential effects of transdermal estradiol and sequential progestagens on impedance to flow within the uterine arteries of postmenopausal women. *Fertil. Steril.*, **58**, 959–63

26. Weiner, Z., Beck, D., Rottem, S., Brandes, J. M. and Thaler, I. (1993). Uterine artery flow velocity waveforms and color flow imaging in women with perimenopausal and postmenopausal bleeding. *Acta Obstet. Gynecol. Scand.*, **72**, 162–6

27. Kurjak, A. and Zalud, I. (1991). The characterization of uterine tumors by transvaginal color Doppler. *Ultrasound Obstet. Gyencol.*, **1**, 50–2

28. Kurjak, A., Kupesic-Urek, S. and Miric, D. (1992). The assessment of benign uterine tumor vascularization by transvaginal color Doppler. *Ultrasound Med. Biol.*, **18**, 645–9

29. Kurjak, A., Salihagic, A., Kupesic-Urek, S. and Predanic, A. (1992). Clinical value of the assessment of gynaecological tumor angiogenesis by transvaginal colour Doppler. *Ann. Med.*, **24**, 97–103

30. Carter, J. R., Lau, M., Saltzman, A. K., Hartenbach, E. M., Chen, M. D., Johnson, P. R., Fowler, J. M., Carlson, J. W., Carson, L. F. and Twiggs, L. B. (1994). Gray scale and color flow Doppler characterization of uterine tumors. *J. Ultrasound Med.*, **13**, 835–40

31. Kurjak, A., Kupesic, S., Shalan, H., Jukic, S., Kosuta, D. and Ilias, M. (1995). Uterine sarcoma: a report of 10 cases studied by transvaginal color and pulsed Doppler sonography. *Gynecol. Oncol.*, **59**, 342–6

32. Sladkevicius, P., Valentin, L. and Marsal, K. (1996). Transvaginal Doppler examination of uteri with myomas. *J. Clin. Ultrasound*, **24**, 135–40

33. Sosic, A., Skupski, D. W., Streltzoff, J., Yun, H. and Chervenak, F. A. (1996). Vascularity of uterine myomas: assessment by color and pulsed Doppler ultrasound. *Int. J. Gynecol. Obstet.*, **54**, 245–50

34. Butram, V. and Reiter, R. (1981). Uterine leiomyomata: etiology, symptomatology, and management. *Fertil. Steril.*, **36**, 433–45

35. Schwartz, L. B., Diamond, M. P. and Schwartz, P. E. (1993). Leiomyosarcoma: clinical presentation. *Am. J. Obstet. Gynecol.*, **168**, 180–3

36. Filicori, M., Hall, D. A., Loughlin, J. S., Vale, W. and Crowley, W. F. (1983). A conservative approach to the management of uterine leiomyomata: pituitary desensitization by a luteinising hormone releasing hormone analogue. *Am. J. Obstet. Gynecol.*, **147**, 726–7

37. Friedman, A. J. (1993). Use of gonadotropin-releasing hormone agonists before myomectomy. *Clin. Obstet. Gynecol.*, **36**, 650–9

38. Stovall, T. G., Summit, R. L., Washburn, S. A. and Ling, F. W. (1994). Gonadotropin-releasing agonist use before hysterectomy. *Am. J. Obstet. Gynecol.*, **170**, 1744–51

39. Matta, W. H. M., Stabile, I., Shaw, R. W. and Campbell, S. (1988). Doppler assessment of uterine blood flow changes in patients with fibroids receiving the gonadotropin-releasing hormone agonist buserelin. *Fertil. Steril.*, **49**, 1083–5

40. Creighton, S., Bourne, T. H., Lawton, F. G., Crayford, T. J. B., Vyas, S., Campbell, S. *et al.* (1994). Use of transvaginal ultrasonography with color Doppler imaging to determine an appropriate treatment regimen for uterine fibroids with a GnRH agonist before surgery: a preliminary study. *Ultrasound Obstet. Gynecol.*, **4**, 494–8

Uterine sarcoma

12

S. Kupesic and A. Kurjak

INTRODUCTION

Uterine sarcoma is a rare tumor, accounting for only 1–3% of all female genital tract malignancy and between 3 and 7.4% of malignant tumors of the corpus uteri[1]. It is a unique tumor because it is both rare and characterized by extremely aggressive behavior, which leads to an early pattern of widespread dissemination and death[2]. Through the years, several questions regarding these tumors have remained unanswered, and a method for its early and correct diagnosis is still unknown. Furthermore, uterine sarcoma is expected to be more common in the near future, as gynecologists are gaining familiarity with the conservative treatment of uterine myomas[3,4].

Sarcomas of the uterus are morphologically and histologically heterogenous tumors that have a much poorer prognosis than endometrial carcinoma; the 5-year survival rate is reported to be about 49% for uterine sarcomas compared with about 87% for endometrial carcinomas[5,6]. The annual incidence of uterine sarcomas in the USA has been reported as 17.1 per million; most were mixed mesodermal sarcomas (48%) and leiomyosarcomas (37%)[6,7].

The results of studies of risk factors showed an increased incidence in women receiving therapeutic ionizing radiation[8]. Harlow and colleagues[9] reported a 27-fold and 60% increased risk of malignant Müllerian sarcoma and leiomyosarcoma among black women compared with white women.

It seems that early onset on menses (before the age of 13) was associated with an increased risk of leiomyosarcoma, while lower risk was noted among parous women[6]. The risk further decreased with increasing number of live births.

HISTOLOGICAL TYPES OF UTERINE SARCOMA

Uterine sarcomas may be divided into those arising from the myometrium (leiomyosarcomas) or endometrial stroma (endometrial stromal sarcomas) and those with an epithelial component (malignant mixed Müllerian tumors and adenosarcomas)[6].

Careful preservation of the specimen and careful examination of the sectioned material is required at histopathology.

Leiomyosarcoma

Leiomyosarcomas represent one-third of uterine sarcomas and are composed of smooth muscle[10]. Mitotic index, cytological atypia and coagulative tumor cell necrosis are histological parameters that predict the nature and behavior of the smooth muscle tumor[11].

Endometrial stromal sarcomas

Endometrial stromal sarcomas (ESS) are divided into two subtypes[6]: low-grade ESS and high-grade ESS. Low-grade ESS are composed of cells mimicking the proliferative endometrial stromal cells that infiltrate the endometrium, whereas high-grade ESS have no specific features, but an infiltrating pattern suggests an origin from endometrial stromal cells.

Malignant mixed Müllerian tumors

Malignant mixed Müllerian tumors are the most common sarcomas of the uterus. They contain malignant epithelial and stromal elements, and are subdivided into homogeneous and heterogeneous subtypes according to the origin of the sarcomatous elements[6]. The fibrosarcoma is the most homogeneous, and the rhabdomyosarcoma the most heterogeneous component.

The endometrial component has been shown to be the element with the greatest impact on the tumor's behavior. The prognosis and survival rates are dependent on the spread of the tumor and its metastatic potential. However, an overall low survival rate (20%) is a main characteristic of this sarcoma type[6].

Adenosarcomas

Adenosarcoma contains a benign epithelial component and a malignant stromal component. According to the ratio of these, the prognosis for this group of patients is more or less favorable.

CLINICAL PRESENTATION

Abnormal vaginal bleeding is the most common presenting symptom in patients with uterine sarcoma. Lower abdominal pain or pressure and palpable abdominal mass are additional findings. An enlarged bulky uterus is palpated, and tumor may be seen protruding through the cervix, particularly in patients with mixed Müllerian tumor[6,12]. Dilatation and currettage may be helpful in distinguishing benign from malignant pathology only if the tumor is submucosal.

Some studies have shown that the mean age of patients with sarcoma is nearly a decade older than the mean age of patients with leiomyomas[13,14]. Clinically, a rapid increase in the size of a uterine tumor after menopause arouses suspicion of sarcoma[14]. The signs and symptoms that occur in women with leiomyomas are also produced by sarcomas.

ULTRASOUND AND COLOR DOPPLER IMAGING

Transvaginal ultrasonography is a non-invasive technique, highly accepted by patients, which affords detailed delineation of the uterus, its myometrium and main uterine vessels. However, even the currently available transvaginal probes have not improved the ability of this technique to distinguish between leiomyoma and sarcoma.

Most of the leiomyosarcomas are solitary and intramural. They have an average size of 10 cm and poorly defined margins. Sarcomas tend to be larger and softer than leiomyomas, and they have irregular margins and more pronounced vascularization, hemorrhage and necrosis. The introduction of color and pulsed Doppler imaging allows non-invasive study of normal and abnormal vasculature and helps to differentiate between benign and malignant tumors *in vivo*[15-21].

Kurjak and co-workers[22] analyzed ten cases of uterine sarcoma by transvaginal color and pulsed Doppler (Table 1). Doppler sonographic patterns were compared with 150 normal and 1850 myomatous uteri. In this study blood flow indices of primary vessels (uterine artery) and secondary vessels (intratumoral neovasculariza-

Table 1 Clinical, pathological and blood flow characteristics in ten uterine sarcomas

Case	Symptom	Age (years)	Pathology	FIGO stage	RI
1	Mass	17*	sarcoma botrioides	IV	0.33
2	Bleeding	55	leiomyosarcoma	I	0.32
3	Bleeding	44*	leiomyosarcoma	I	0.39
4	Bleeding	60	leiomyosarcoma	III	0.35
5	Pain	59	leiomyosarcoma	II	0.42
6	Bleeding	64	leiomyosarcoma	III	0.37
7	Bleeding	58	leiomyosarcoma	III	0.38
8	Bleeding	62	endometrial stromal sarcoma	IV	0.40
9	Bleeding	65	leiomyosarcoma	III	0.37
10	Bleeding	41*	leiomyosarcoma	I	0.33

*Premenopausal women

Table 2 Resistance index (RI) of the myometrial vessels in studied groups

	n	Visualization rate		RI	
		n	%	Mean	SD
Normal uterus	150	63	42	0.68[*‡]	0.02
Myomatous uterus	1850	1221	66	0.54[*†]	0.12
Sarcomatous uterus	10	10	100	0.37[†‡]	0.03

[*]$p < 0.05$; [†]$p < 0.001$; [‡]$p < 0.001$

Table 3 Uterine artery resistance index (RI) in relation to histopathological findings

	n	Uterine artery RI	
		Mean	SD
Normal uterus	150	0.88[*‡]	0.09
Myomatous uterus	1850	0.74[*†]	0.08
Sarcomatous uterus	10	0.62[†‡]	0.07

[*]$p < 0.05$; [†]$p < 0.001$; [‡]$p < 0.001$

tion) were assessed. All cases of uterine sarcoma (100%) revealed abnormal tumoral blood vessels. The typical finding in sarcoma was the presence of irregular, thin and randomly dispersed vessels in the peripheral and/or central area of the tumor (Figures 1 and 2), with very low impedance shunts (mean resistance index (RI) = 0.37 ± 0.03) (Figures 3 and 4; Table 2). The RI ranged from 0.32 to 0.42, which was significantly lower than that of normal and myomatous uteri ($p < 0.001$). There was no significant difference between the RI in the right and left uterine arteries in each separate group; however, there was a decline in these values from normal, through myomatosis, to sarcomatous uteri. In the group of patients with sarcoma, both uterine arteries showed a low RI, (0.62 ± 0.07) in comparison with that of normal (0.88 ± 0.09) or myomatous uteri (0.74 ± 0.08) in women matched for age and parity (Table 3). However, one patient with uterine leiomyosarcoma showed a slightly increasing intratumoral RI value (0.42) and was shown as a false negative. Using a cut-off point of 0.40 for the RI, the authors were able to distinguish between benign and malignant myometrial tumors with a sensitivity of 90.91%, specificity of 99.82%, positive predictive value of 71.43% and negative predictive value of 99.96%.

Our previous study[19] demonstrated that the vascularization of the benign uterine masses is largely dependent on the tumor size, its position and the extent of secondary degenerative changes (Figure 5). The vascularization of leiomyoma is supported by pre-existing myometrial vessels originating from terminal branches of the uterine artery. A leiomyoma grows centripetally as proliferations of smooth muscle cells and fibrous connective tissue, creating a pseudocapsule of compressed muscle fibers. Therefore, color Doppler demonstrates most of the color leiomyometrial vessels at its periphery. In most cases peripheral blood vessels encircling the leiomyoma are dilated veins (Figures 6 and 7), whereas those 'perforating' the peripheral part are usually arteries (Figure 8). The mean RI of the myometrial blood flow in patients with leiomyoma in this study was 0.54, and the mean PI was 0.89.

Large and laterally positioned leiomyomas, especially those with necrosis and inflammatory changes, may show an increased diastolic flow and, consequently, a low RI. It seems clear from conflicting Doppler data that differences and improvements in instrument design have made smaller vessels more visible. Seeing smaller vessels has led to the recognition of occasional low-resistance vessels in benign growths. Biological variations dictate that all malignant growths may not have vessels, particularly if growth has stabilized or if there is no metastatic potential. We have demonstrated an overlap between four cases of uterine myomas and uterine sarcomas in terms of an RI cut-off point of 0.40. This observation awaits further studies, as it could be due to the rapid rate of growth of such a myoma or due to a premalignant state.

Hata and colleagues[23] retrospectively analyzed 41 patients with histologically proven

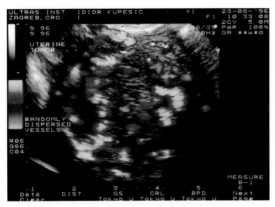

Figure 1 Randomly dispersed, newly formed vessels demonstrated by color Doppler imaging in a case of uterine sarcoma

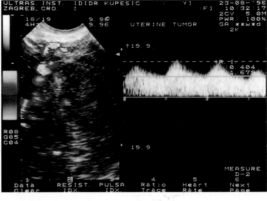

Figure 3 Irregular vascular network demonstrated within the heterogeneous uterine tumor (left). Pulsed Doppler analysis shows a low resistance index (RI = 0.40) (right)

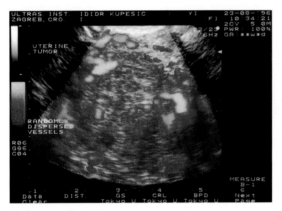

Figure 2 The same patient as in Figure 1. Power Doppler imaging facilitates the visualization of small, randomly dispersed vessels

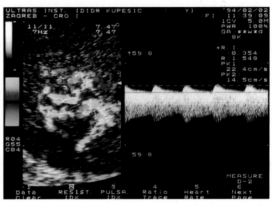

Figure 4 Transvaginal color Doppler scan of a small heterogeneous nodule in a postmenopausal patient (left). The pulsed Doppler waveform analysis extracted from the 'hot area' (right) demonstrates low-resistance flow (RI = 0.35) typical of uterine malignancy

uterine leiomyoma and five with uterine sarcoma (four leiomyosarcomas and one mixed mesodermal tumor). The parameters analyzed were peak systolic velocity (PSV) and RI. The authors found no significant difference between the RI in the uterine leiomyomas (0.64 ± 0.11) and the uterine sarcomas (0.63 ± 0.18). However, the PSV was significantly higher in the uterine sarcomas (71.0 ± 31.7) than in the uterine leiomyomas (22.7 ± 9.2) ($p < 0.05$). When a cut-off value for the PSV of 41 cm/s was considered, the detection rate for uterine sarcoma was 80.0% and the false-positive rate was

2.4%. However, the small number of the patients and the usage of an angle-dependent Doppler parameter such as PSV are the main objections to the study.

It can be postulated that leiomyosarcomas arise *de novo* in most cases, but some are thought to arise from the malignant transformation of a leiomyoma. In many cases gross pathology cannot distinguish a leiomyosarcoma from a leiomyoma with degeneration and irregular borders. Sometimes only a high mitotic count can distinguish sarcomas from cellular myomas[24,25]. During a 1-year prospective study by

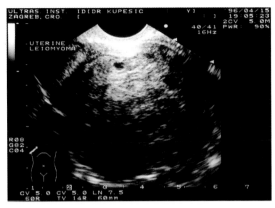

Figure 5 Huge, heterogeneous uterine tumor with areas of cystic degeneration and necrosis

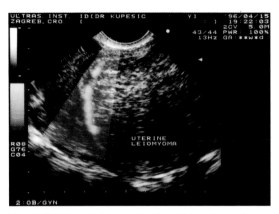

Figure 7 Regularly separated peripheral vessels in a patient with uterine leiomyoma as shown by power Doppler imaging

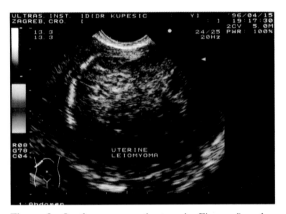

Figure 6 In the same patient as in Figure 5, color Doppler imaging demonstrates a thick vessel encircling the leiomyoma

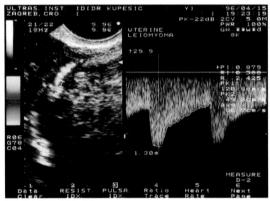

Figure 8 Waveform analysis (right) indicates the high velocity (120.8 cm/s) and moderate resistance of the tumor blood flow (RI = 0.59) in a patient with uterine leiomyoma

Kurjak and associates[22], transvaginal color Doppler detected one uterine sarcoma with a low RI value (0.33), which fell into a borderline category. Microscopic pathology detected five mitoses per high-powered field (HPF) and moderate cellular atypia. Other sarcomas were characterized by moderate to marked cellular atypia and a mitotic rate in excess of 10 mitotic figures/10 HPF. Moreover, some myomas showed infiltration of the myometrium and cellular pleomorphism, albeit usually not to the degree seen in leiomyosarcoma. It should be concluded that a careful transvaginal color Doppler examination of uterine tumor should include morphological changes and analysis of vascularization (brightness of color, vascular location and type of vascularization). Malignant uterine masses display bright color signals from randomly dispersed vessels, while pulsed Doppler analysis demonstrates low vascular impedance. In huge and necrotic leiomyomas, areas of neovascularization within the central parts usually demonstrate low vascular resistance due to the release of vasoactive compounds, whereas a peripheral ring of angiogenesis is characterized by moderate impedance to blood flow. It seems that the uterine artery vascular impedance quality measured by RI can be used as an additional parameter in the diagnosis of leiomyosarcoma, since the RI shows significantly lower values when compared to that of uterine leiomyoma.

Because of their rarity, uterine sarcomas are not suitable for screening[6]. Bimanual examination is unlikely to detect an early disease, and dilatation and curettage (D&C) procedures should detect only lesions originating from or invading into the endometrium. Transvaginal ultrasound can detect differences in myometrial tissue density, and therefore can be used for detection of uterine sarcoma. Because of low specificity this method is not appropriate as a screening procedure. Similar specificities have been obtained by magnetic resonance imaging (MRI). However, such an evaluation requires at least a few high-resolution images, sample time and huge expense. A method that can target patients at risk for uterine sarcoma should be non-invasive, less expensive, easily repeatable and reproducible.

Vascularization of the uterine tumors, if used together with analysis of morphology and size, can increase our accuracy in differentiation between uterine sarcoma and leiomyoma. However, it is unrealistic to expect Doppler studies to clarify confounding histological findings. It seems that the multiparameter sonographic approach, which includes morphology and size depicted by transvaginal ultrasonography and color flow imaging with pulsed Doppler analysis of neovascular signals, can help in diagnosis of uterine sarcoma in high-risk groups such as postmenopausal patients with a rapidly enlarging uterus. Therefore, serial measurements are recommended for evaluation of the myometrial density, follow-up of the tumoral growth, and detection of the impedance to blood flow. Only such complex observations can lead to proper diagnosis of these rare tumors with unpredictable prognosis.

References

1. Olah, K. S., Gee, H., Blunt, S., Dunn, J. A. and Chan, K. K. (1991). Retrospective analysis of 318 cases of uterine sarcoma. *Eur. J. Cancer*, **27**, 1095–9
2. El-Naggar, A. K., Abdul-Karim, F. W., Silva, E. G., McLemore, D. and Garnesy, L. (1991). Uterine stromal neoplasms: a clinicopathologic and DNA flow cytometric correlation. *Hum. Pathol.*, **22**, 897–902
3. Meyer, W. R., Meyer, A. R, Diamond, M. P., Carcangu, M. L., Schwartz, P. E. and DeChernay, A. H. (1990). Unsuspected leiomyosarcoma: treatment with a gonadotropin-releasing hormone analogue. *Obstet. Gynecol.*, **75**, 529–34
4. Berchuck, A., Rubin, S. C. and Hoskins, W. J. (1990). Treatment of endometrial stromal tumors. *Gynecol. Oncol.*, **36**, 60–4
5. Czesnin, K. and Wronkovski, Z. (1978). Second malignancies of the irradiated area in patients treated for uterine cervix cancer. *Gynecol. Oncol.*, **6**, 309–14
6. Levenback, C. F., Tortolero, L. G., Pandey, D. K., Malpica, A., Baker, V. V., Whittaker, L., Johnson, E. and Follen Mitchell, M. (1996). Uterine sarcoma. In Follen Mitchell, M., Schot-

tenfeld, D. and Kitlong, W. (eds.) *Obstetrics and Gynecology Clinics of North America: Gynecologic Cancer Prevention*, Vol. 23, pp. 457–73. (Philadelphia: WB Saunders)
7. Page, H. S. and Asire, A. J. (1985). *Cancer Rates and Risks*. NIH publication no. 85–691. (Washington, DC: US Department of Health and Human Services)
8. Schwartz, Z., Dgani, R., Lancet, M. and Kesser, I. (1985). Uterine sarcoma in Israel: a study of 104 cases. *Gynecol. Oncol.*, **20**, 354–63
9. Harlow, B. L., Weiss, N. S. and Lofton, S. (1986). The epidemiology of sarcomas of the uterus. *J. Natl. Cancer Inst.*, **76**, 399–402
10. Zalovdek, C. and Norris, H. J. (1994). Mesenchymal tumors of the uterus. In Kurman, R. J. (ed.) *Blanstein's Pathology of the Female Genital Tract*, 4th edn., pp. 487–95. (New York: Spinger Verlag)
11. Bell, S. W., Kempson, R. L. and Hendricson, M. R. (1994). Problematic uterine smooth muscle neoplasms. A clinicopathologic study of 213 cases. *Am. J. Surg. Pathol.*, **18**, 535–58
12. Dinh, T. V., Slavin, R. E., Bhagavan, B. J., Hannigan, E. V., Tiamson, E. M. and Yandell, R. B. (1989). Mixed mullerian tumors of the uterus:

a clinicopathologic study. *Obstet. Gynecol.*, **74**, 388–92

13. Marchese, M. J., Liskow, A. S. and Crum, C. P. (1984). Uterine sarcomas: a clinicopathologic study, 1965–1981. *Gynecol. Oncol.*, **18**, 299–304

14. Christopherson, W. M., Williamson, E. O. and Gray, L. A. (1972). Leiomyosarcoma of the uterus. *Cancer*, **29**, 1512–16

15. Kurjak, A. and Zalud, I. (1991). The characterization of uterine tumors by transvaginal color Doppler. *Ultrasound Obstet. Gynecol.*, **1**, 50–2

16. Hata, T., Hata, K., Senoh, D., Makihara, K., Aoki, S., Takamiya, D. and Kitao, M. (1989). Doppler ultrasound assessment of tumor vascularity in gynecologic disorders. *J. Ultrasound Med.*, **8**, 309–13

17. Kurjak, A., Shalan, H., Kupesic, S., Predanic, M., Zalud, I., Breyer, B. and Jukic, S. (1993). Transvaginal color Doppler sonography in the assessment of pelvic tumor vascularity. *Ultrasound Obstet. Gynecol.*, **3**, 1–15

18. Bourne, T. H. (1991). Transvaginal color Doppler in gynecology. *Ultrasound Obstet. Gynecol.*, **1**, 359–73

19. Kurjak, A., Kupesic-Urek, S. and Miric, D. (1992). The assessment of benign uterine tumors by transvaginal color Doppler. *Ultrasound Med. Biol.*, **18**, 645–9

20. Kurjak, A., Shalan, H., Sosic, A., Benic, S., Zudenigo, D. and Kupesic, S. (1993). Endometrial carcinoma in postmenopausal women. Evaluation by transvaginal color Doppler sonography. *Am. J. Obstet. Gynecol.*, **6**, 1597–603

21. Kurjak, A. and Kupesic, S. (1995). Transvaginal color Doppler and pelvic tumor vascularity – lessons learned and future challenges. *J. Ultrasound Obstet. Gynecol.*, **6**, 145–59

22. Kurjak, A., Kupesic, S., Shalan, H., Jukic, S., Kosuta, D. and Ilijas, M. (1995). Uterine sarcoma: a report of 10 cases studied by transvaginal color and pulsed Doppler sonography. *Gynecol. Oncol.*, **59**, 342–6

23. Hata, K., Hata, T., Marayama, R. and Hirai, M. (1997). Uterine sarcoma: can it be differentiated from uterine leiomyoma with Doppler ultrasonography? A preliminary report. *Ultrasound Obstet. Gynecol.*, **9**, 101–4

24. Burns, B., Curry, H. R. and Bell, M. E. A. (1979). Morphologic features of prognostic significance in uterine smooth muscle tumors: a review of eighty-four cases. *Am. J. Obstet. Gynecol.*, **135**, 109–14

25. Ezra, J., Fields, S. and Kopolovic, J. (1988). Benign uterine leiomyoma suspected of sarcomatous change on an ultrasound scan and computerized topography. *Arch. Gynecol. Obstet.*, **241**, 255–8

Doppler ultrasound and hormonal replacement therapy

13

I. Žalud and H. Schulman

INTRODUCTION

Menopause is defined as the permanent cessation of menses. This is only one aspect of the climacteric, during which time women undergo endocrine, somatic and psychological changes that span several years. Because these changes are related both to aging and to estrogen depletion, it is difficult to quantify the respective effects of each. The mean age of women at menopause is 51 years; approximately 4% of women undergo a natural menopause before 40 years of age. The age at which menopause occurs is not influenced by prolonged periods of hypothalamic amenorrhea, number of pregnancies or oral contraceptive use. Although life expectancy has risen considerably during the 20th century, the average age at menopause has not changed since antiquity. Therefore, women in industrialized countries today will live one-third of their lifespan after ovarian failure. The age at which the menopause occurs is genetically predetermined, unlike the age of menarche, which is related to body mass. The only environmental factor affecting the age at menopause is cigarette smoking, which decreases the age at menopause by about 2 years.

The aging process of the ovary appears to begin during fetal development. Although 7 million oogonia are present at 20 weeks' gestation, only 700 000 remain at birth. Following birth, the number of oocytes continues to decline, even before the onset of puberty. For several years prior to menopause, estradiol and progesterone production decline, despite the occurrence of ovulatory cycles. This waning of ovarian follicular activity reduces the negative feedback inhibition of estradiol on the hypothalamic–pituitary system, resulting in a gradual rise in the concentration of follicle stimulating hormone (FSH). The remaining ovarian follicles are increasingly those which are less responsive to FSH, and menopause occurs when the residual follicles are refractory to elevated concentrations of FSH.

After the menopause, ovarian production of estrogen ceases and circulating levels fall dramatically, with estrone levels becoming greater than estradiol levels. Extraglandular conversion of circulating androstenedione accounts for almost all estrone production. After the menopause, about 85% of androstenedione comes from adrenal secretion and about 15% from the ovaries. The conversion of androstenedione to estrone takes place mainly in the fatty tissue; therefore, obese women have higher levels of estrone and are less likely to be estrogen-deficient.

About one-third of a woman's life is now after the menopause. Estrogen replacement therapy can alleviate hot flushes and night sweats, relieve vaginal atrophy, prevent bone loss and osteoporotic features, reduce the risk of cardiovascular disease and decrease overall mortality in postmenopausal women. Hormone replacement therapy (HRT) may also increase the risk of endometrial and breast cancers.

Prospective studies suggest that HRT users have a longer life expectancy than non-users[1–3]. The evidence strongly indicates that overall mortality is reduced 20–50% among HRT users. Handerson and colleagues[1] observed that women who had used estrogen had a 20% lower mortality from all causes; those who had taken HRT for at least 15 years or were current users had a 30–40% lower mortality rate. This chapter deals with the benefits and risks of HRT and how Doppler ultrasound can help in the management of menopause.

CLINICAL ASPECTS

Decreasing estrogen production leads to atrophy of the vagina, which can produce the distressful symptoms of senile vaginitis or atrophic vaginitis. This type of vaginitis can cause itching, burning, discomfort, dyspareunia and also vaginal bleeding when the epithelium thins. Senile vaginitis is best treated with estrogen replacement therapy. Local therapy can be used for the first few weeks. However, because vaginal administration of estrogen results in irregular systemic absorption, for long-term prevention of vaginal atrophy as well as osteoporosis, the patient is best treated with systemic estrogen. Estrogen deprivation may also cause the structures that support the uterus – the cardinal and uterosacral ligaments – to lose their tonicity, and uterine descensus may occur.

The trigone of the bladder and the urethra is embryologically derived from estrogen-dependent tissue, and estrogen deficiency can lead to their atrophy, producing symptoms of urinary urgency, incontinence, dysuria and urinary frequency. Another problem that can develop with decreased circulating estrogen levels is decreased synthesis of collagen, which forms the connective tissue beneath the vaginal epithelium. This change may decrease the support of the posterior urethrovesicle angle, and urinary stress incontinence can develop. Loss of collagen can also lead to dynamically symptomatic cystoceles and/or rectoceles. These urinary symptoms can be alleviated or prevented by estrogen replacement therapy.

The pathognomonic symptom of menopause is the hot flush, which is caused by a decrease in circulating estrogen levels. The change in estrogen levels leads to alterations in the hypothalamus that are probably mediated through the central nervous system. When the change in estrogen levels is not gradual but sudden, such as occurs after premenopausal oophorectomy, the individual is more likely to develop symptomatic hot flushes.

About 75% of all women going through menopause develop hot flushes. Obese individuals are less likely to develop flushes, as they do not have as great a decrease in estrogen levels. About one-third of women with hot flushes have sufficiently severe symptoms to require medical assistance. About one-half of the patients with flushes have at least one a day, and about 20% have more than one a day. These flushes frequently occur at night, awaken the individual and then produce insomnia. Hot flushes do not persist in most women for more than 2–3 years, and it is uncommon for a woman to have hot flushes more than 5 years after menopause.

The most effective treatment for the hot flush is estrogen. Since so many of the hot flushes occur at night, it is advisable for the patient to ingest the estrogen tablet before bedtime. Some patients, such as those with a history of cancer of the breast or recent (< 2 years) cancer of the endometrium, should not take estrogen. The next best therapy is a progestogen. Oral medroxyprogesterone acetate (MPA) at a dose of 20 mg/day relieves hot flushes significantly more effectively than placebo. Unfortunately, MPA does not prevent vaginal or urethral atrophy, but it will diminish hot flushes in patients who cannot take estrogen. Injections of Depo-Provera® (DMPA) at a dose of 150 mg once every 3 months relieve hot flushes very well. Other agents shown to reduce hot flushes significantly include clonidine, naloxone and methyldopa (Aldomet®), but these drugs are not usually prescribed for this purpose.

Symptoms such as anxiety, depression, irritability and fatigue increase after menopause. Several studies have demonstrated that estrogen improves many of these psychological symptoms significantly better than placebo, particularly depression, in addition to relieving the hot flush and allowing the patient to sleep better. Postmenopausal estrogen users have significantly thicker skin and a greater amount of collagen in the dermis than those not using estrogen. Systemic estrogen use can retard wrinkling and thinning of the skin postmenopausally.

RISK CONSIDERATIONS

Many epidemiological studies have reported that there is significantly increased risk of endometrial hyperplasia developing in postmenopausal women who are ingesting estrogen without progestins, compared with those not using estrogen. The risk increases with increasing duration of use of estrogen as well as with increasing dosage. The endometrial cancer that develops in estrogen users is nearly always well-differentiated and is usually cured by a simple hysterectomy. The risk of developing endometrial carcinoma in women receiving estrogen replacement can be markedly reduced by taking progestogens. The duration of progestin therapy is more important than the dosage. The use of progestins may lower the chances of postmenopausal estrogen users developing cancer of the endometrium, and therefore progestins should be given to postmenopausal women receiving estrogen if they have a uterus. The addition of a progestin to estrogen therapy does not appear to cause an increase of any other systemic disease and acts synergistically with estrogen to cause a slight increase in bone density. The use of synthetic progestins, however, may reverse the beneficial effect of estrogen upon serum lipids.

The first reports of case–control studies showing increased risk for endometrial cancer in postmenopausal women taking estrogen replacement therapy (ERT) appeared in 1981[4]. The studies also showed that the risk of endometrial cancer increased with higher doses and longer duration of ERT. Women using ERT for 5 years or more have about a five- to tenfold increased risk compared to never-users of ERT. Although these estrogen-induced tumors are usually at an early stage and minimally invasive at diagnosis, an increased risk of disseminated endometrial cancer has been documented[5,6]. Recent studies highlight the fact that the increased risk of endometrial cancer remains up to 15 years after discontinuation of therapy[7,8]. Therefore, patients who have received ERT require careful post-treatment surveillance. As we will see later in this chapter, ultrasound can help to reduce the risk of endometrial carcinoma.

Evidence is inconsistent regarding the association between ERT and breast cancer. Recent reviews and meta-analysis of the epidemiological studies of estrogen and breast cancer suggest that a low dose (< 0.625 mg) and/or shorter (< 5 years) use of HRT do not substantially increase the risk of breast cancer[9].

The epidemiological data showing a reduction in heart attacks in estrogen users were derived from women taking estrogen without a progestin. Whether the addition of a progestin to the regimen will reverse the beneficial action of estrogen upon cardiovascular disease remains to be determined. Nevertheless, it would appear prudent to use the lowest doses of progestin that will prevent the endometrial proliferation produced by estrogen.

TREATMENT REGIMENS

Estrogen therapy for postmenopausal women should be given in the lowest possible dose that relieves vasomotor symptoms, prevents vaginal–urethral epithelial atrophy, maintains the collagen content of the skin, reduces the rate of bone resorption and prevents acceleration of atherosclerosis. Estrogen therapy given to postmenopausal women should result in physiological and not pharmacological circulating levels of estrogen, so that the risks of hypertension and thromboembolic disease are not increased. This dose of estrogen, termed the physiological replacement, is 0.625 mg of conjugated equine estrogens or estrogen sulfate or 1 mg of micronized estradiol. The long-term effects of transdermal estradiol have not yet been determined, but it appears that the 0.05-mg skin patch provides physiological estrogen replacement. Higher doses of estrogen may be needed for 1 or 2 years to relieve hot flushes. Vaginal administration of estrogen may be used initially to relieve atrophic vaginitis but it is best to employ other routes for long-term use as vaginal estrogen absorption is greatly variable.

If progestin is added to the regimen in order to protect the endometrium, it does not negate the beneficial effects of estrogen on vasomotor symptoms or on bone density. The progestin may have an adverse effect on the vaginal and urethral mucosa, and may produce undesired central nervous system symptoms and adversely affect mood and the sense of well-being. Depending on the dose and biological activity of the specific progestin, the favorable anti-atherogenic lipid profile produced by estrogen may also be altered, and therefore may possibly result in a partial or complete loss of the cardio-vascular protective effect of unopposed estrogen. The epidemiological studies showing a reduction in myocardial infarction with hormonal replacement looked at only groups of women taking estrogen alone, without progestins. Finally, a hormonal regimen should be selected that produces the least amount of uterine bleeding, and the bleeding should occur at regular intervals. One of the primary reasons that post-menopausal women decide not to use estrogen, or discontinue its use, is the occurrence of uterine bleeding. For this reason, combination instead of sequential estrogen–progestin regimens are being increasingly prescribed, as the former regimen may be associated with no bleeding after the first few months.

The benefit of including a progestin in the estrogen replacement regimen is protection of the endometrium. Unfortunately, this benefit is accompanied by an increase in central nervous system symptoms and changes in mood and sense of well-being. Women who have undergone a hysterectomy are no longer at risk for endometrial cancer. Until other significant benefits of progestin therapy for menopausal women are established, an unopposed estrogen regimen, cyclic or continuous, is recommended for postmenopausal women who no longer have a uterus. For postmenopausal women who have not had a hysterectomy, there are many treatment regimens used, in addition to the combined continuous estrogen–progestin regimens. An estrogen-only regimen may be utilized to optimize protection from cardiovascular disease, in conjunction with an annual endometrial biopsy or vaginal ultrasonography to measure the endometrial thickness.

Several investigators have shown that the women with endometrial thickness of 5 mm or less measured by ultrasound had a histological diagnosis of atrophic endometrium[10,11]. This technique may therefore be used instead of annual biopsy to screen postmenopausal women with a uterus receiving estrogen without a progestin or those who bleed with a continuous combined estrogen–progestin regimen. Currently in clinical practice, physicians most often include a progestin in the hormonal replacement regimen of postmenopausal women who have a uterus. Various regimens, both sequential and continuous combined, have been utilized. The hormones are usually administered in a cyclic manner, with a daily dose of estrogen given the first 25 days each month and a daily dose of progestin administered concomitantly with the last 10–14 days of the estrogen. The estrogen may also be given every day of the month in a continuous fashion and the progestin given daily for the first 10–14 days of the month with the combined regimen. The latter sequential regimen is easier for patients to remember than the former. With the continuous combined regimen, both the estrogen and the progestin are administered every day of the month or 5 out of 7 days each week. The cyclic regimens usually result in monthly withdrawal bleeding, which may lessen with continued use. The continuous regimen may result in breakthrough bleeding during the first few months, but with longer use nearly all women remain amenorrheic. Because endogenous fluctuating estrogen levels in the early menopause may contribute to uterine bleeding with the continuous combined regimen, it has been recommended that the sequential regimen be used in the first 5 years after the menopause, after which the combined regimen can be utilized to increase patient compliance.

The minimal dosage and type of progestin necessary to prevent endometrial cancer have not been determined. For postmenopausal women receiving 0.625 mg of conjugated equine estrogens, 2.5 mg of medroxyprogesterone acetate reduced nuclear and cytosol estrogen receptor levels to those found before estrogen administration. Since the side-effects of progestin therapy are dose-related, reduction in dose of progestin to the minimum that still protects the endometrium may lead to improved patient compliance. Therefore, although 10 mg of medroxyprogesterone acetate is usually presented in the sequential regimen, only 2.5 mg is needed when given continuously, to prevent endometrial hyperplasia.

A routine pretreatment endometrial biopsy is unnecessary, as it is not cost-effective. Also, routine annual biopsies are not necessary. If breakthrough bleeding occurs, and if ultrasonography shows the endometrial thickness to be > 5 mm, then therapy can be stopped for a few weeks to see if the endometrium shrinks. Annual mammography should be recommended for all women aged 50 years or older, regardless of whether they are on estrogen therapy, as the incidence of breast cancer steadily increases as a woman ages. Contraindications to estrogen therapy occur infrequently. These include a history of breast cancer and thromboembolic disease associated with oral contraceptive use or pregnancy. There are no data to support these contraindications, and the American College of Obstetricians and Gynecologists issued a committee opinion in 1991 stating that clinicians may elect to prescribe estrogen replacement to women with a past history of breast cancer who wish to receive the benefits of estrogen. Alternatively, progestins or clonidine can be given to reduce hot flushes and a vaginal lubricant given to relieve the symptoms of vaginal atrophy. The Centers for Disease Control have reported that women with a positive family history of breast cancer involving either a second-degree or a first- degree relative may use estrogen replacement therapy without an increased risk of breast cancer. Women with active liver disease should avoid the oral administration of estrogen.

Estrogen is the treatment of choice for the relief of vasomotor symptoms and symptoms caused by vaginal and urethral mucosa atrophy. In addition, estrogen therapy maintains the integument, improves mood, prevents postmenopausal osteoporosis and, above all, significantly reduces the morbidity and mortality associated with cardiovascular disease. Nearly all postmenopausal women can derive a substantial benefit from the use of estrogen replacement therapy and several studies have shown that estrogen users have decreased overall mortality compared to women of a similar population who were not taking estrogen[1,2].

PRACTICAL APPROACH

Although menopause is a natural event, and the age of menopause has not changed with time, life expectancy has markedly increased. Therefore it is perhaps 'not natural' for women to be living longer. We have to consider improvements in the quality of a woman's life; fully one-third of a woman's life is spent in an estrogen-deficient state. Often beginning before menopause, symptoms of hot flushes frequently warrant treatment. This may be associated with sometimes subtle but real changes in mood and psychological well-being. Later on, vulvovaginal complaints emerge as an indication for treatment. All these symptoms are pronounced if a woman experiences an abrupt cessation of hormonal function, such as with bilateral oophorectomy. Nevertheless, the primary indications of hormonal replacement are the preventive measures needed to avoid the devastating consequences of osteoporosis and cardiovascular disease. These are late events, however, and preventive strategies of HRT require prolonged use, from the time of menopause, to realize the benefit. Fractures do not usually occur until the sixth decade and myocardial infarction and cardiovascular death usually occur even later, in the seventh decade.

An adequate evaluation of the patient followed by a discussion of the patient's options and her indications for treatment is mandatory. Following this, therapy should be individualized. Flexible prescribing is necessary to meet the needs of all postmenopausal women and at all times during the postmenopausal years. Compliance is major issue that needs to be reinforced. In patient surveys, it has been estimated that most postmenopausal women do not remain on therapy beyond the first 2–3 years. Although fear of cancer, bleeding and other factors are contributory, it was found in patient surveys that the principal reason for noncompliance was the patient not being adequately informed of the real lifelong benefits of estrogen, particularly in terms of osteoporosis prevention and cardiovascular disease. Therefore, a continuous dialog needs to be established between the practitioner and the patient. The goals of this dialog should also include sufficiently flexible prescribing to help with compliance over time. Even if a patient wishes to discontinue treatment and/or to seek alternatives, this important dialog will lead to improved health care for postmenopausal women.

It is important to note that if estrogen is to be prescribed, it should be 'physiological'. Barring the occasional need to increase the dose or modify delivery systems for symptom relief, 17β-estradiol levels should be monitored so that they remain within a range of 40–100 pg/ml. For the prevention of osteoporosis in all women, approximately 50–60 pg/ml of 17β-estradiol is required, although some women require less. Oral estrogens are metabolized to estrone. For convenience, it is appropriate to use oral estrogens as first-line treatment in most circumstances. The choices of using other routes of application include the estradiol patch, transdermal gel, the estradiol subdermal pellet and various vaginal preparations including rings and creams.

Although estrogen remains the mainstay of postmenopausal treatment, HRT usually includes a progestogen in the regimen. Potential concerns with progestogen use are mood disturbances, menstrual bleeding, attenuation of cardiovascular benefits and breast cancer.

The aim of progestogen therapy is to prevent hyperplasia. In order to do this, it is not necessary to induce a full secretory endometrium. Low doses of various progestogens, administered sequentially, such as 2.5 mg medroxyprogesterone acetate, are sufficient to inhibit endometrial estradiol receptors and mitotic activity. It is thus the biochemical machinery, induced by estrogen, and the mitotic activity that have to be inhibited to prevent hyperplasia. A full secretory endometrium is not necessary and the doses that may be required to achieve this may induce unfavorable effects. The practical concern, however, with using low doses of progestogens is cycle control.

DOPPLER ULTRASOUND AND HRT

The endometrial echo in postmenopausal women is generally no more than a thin linear echo generally 1–3 mm in thickness. Postmenopausal bleeding in such patients is usually from an atrophic endometrium. Occasionally, in some postmenopausal patients, the endometrium may not be imaged or may be imaged as an incomplete thin line. This generally reflects an atrophic endometrium.

The influence of HRT on the postmenopausal endometrium has been widely studied[12–16]. Transvaginal ultrasound depicts changes in the endometrial texture and thickness related to the postmenopausal status and hormonal therapy[10,11,17,18]. However, studies of postmenopausal uterine blood flow are not often described. The influence of hormonal therapy and the ageing process on endometrial thickness and uterine artery blood flow needs further attention.

Transvaginal ultrasound makes it possible to show pelvic structures very precisely. As a consequence, subtle changes in endometrium or myometrium can be seen and analyzed more distinctly[19,20]. This is particularly important for women of advanced age now that there is the potential for screening for endometrial cancer[21]. Additionally, with color and pulsed Doppler, it is possible to analyze the quality of blood flow in the uterine artery or any other pelvic vessel[17]. Thus, Doppler adds functional information about morphology obtained with B-mode ultrasound (Figures 1–8).

Recently, we assessed the age and hormonal influence on endometrial and myometrial thickness and uterine blood flow in postmenopausal women[22]. A total of 109 healthy postmenopausal women were examined by transvaginal ultrasonography and color Doppler ultrasonography. Twenty women (18.4%) were under continuous HRT for at least 1 year. In all patients, full thickness of the endometrium and half thickness of the myometrium were measured. Pulsed Doppler waveforms were used to calculate the resistance index for the left and right uterine arteries. Endometrial thickness in the groups without HRT did not change as the years of postmenopause progressed. This was also true for myometrial thickness. The resistance to blood flow in the uterine arteries remained the same as the postmenopause progressed, but with each 5-year analysis, the ability to see the uterine arteries decreased. The duration of the therapy did not affect the measured parameters. The thickness of the endometrium was larger in the groups with HRT in comparison with all groups without HRT ($p < 0.01$). Myometrial thickness and uterine blood flow were not affected and did not show any significant influence from HRT. The conclusion from our study is that continuous hormonal replacement therapy significantly influenced the thickness of postmenopausal endometrium but not myometrium or uterine artery blood flow. Uterine involution is a steady and slow process. Hormonal therapy did not create a significant increase in the number of women with small fibroids.

We observed how continuous hormonal replacement therapy influenced endometrial and myometrial thickness as well as uterine artery blood flow. It is well known that endometrium has hormonal receptors[23]. Hormonal receptors in myometrium or in the wall of uterine vessels have not been extensively studied. Our study shows that hormonal therapy significantly increased the thickness of endometrium ($p < 0.01$) but not the thickness of myometrium, nor uterine blood flow. On the basis of this observation, it might be speculated that the number of hormonal receptors per measurement unit is much higher and/or they are more activated in postmenopausal endometrium in comparison to the myometrium or the peripheral vessel wall. Another possibility is that hormone therapy may be inadequate to affect smooth muscle cells.

The study of Sadan and colleagues[20] showed that in the normal myometrium and fibroids, estrogen receptors act independently at the lower or higher level of the normal serum steroid range. They speculated that it might be an inherent characteristic of fibroids that results in their progressive growth without any abnormal stimulation. This might be partially explained by higher sensitivity and/or a higher

number of active hormonal receptors in fibroma in comparison with normal postmenopausal myometrium. However, small fibroids did not influence any of the measured parameters in our study.

The aging process and its influence on the total size of the uterus have been previously studied[21]. A normal ultrasound appearance of the endometrium in postmenopausal women has been found to exclude endometrial pathology. Endometrial thickness measurement has been introduced as a routine procedure to screen for pathology, especially for endometrial carcinoma. Nasri and co-workers[10] suggested that an endometrial thickness of 5 mm was an appropriate cut-off level for conservative management of patients with postmenopausal bleeding, or in screening for endometrial carcinoma. Varner[14] concluded that, in women with measured endometrial thickness of 5–8 mm, proliferative endometrium could not be distinguished from hyperplastic endometrium or, in one case, low-grade carcinoma. Large polyps and invasive carcinoma with myometrial extension were easily recognized in that study. Endometrial measurement has high sensitivity but very low specificity in screening for endometrial carcinoma. In addition, HRT usually increases endometrial thickness in postmenopausal women. This may result in ambiguous findings when endometrial thickness measurement is used without clinical data.

Our study compared ageing and continuous hormonal influence on the three entities: endometrium, myometrium and uterine blood flow. Although the thickness of endometrium was 0.31 cm in the group of patients with 1–5 years after menopause and 0.23 cm in the group with more than 15 years after menopause, this observation did not reach statistical significance. Since myometrial thickness changes less than endometrial thickness after menopause, this might suggest that changes in postmenopausal endometrium could be more dynamic than in postmenopausal myometrium. This may contribute to abnormal changes such as endometrial cancer. Continuous hormonal therapy influenced the endometrial thickness dramatically but not the normal myometrium. To the

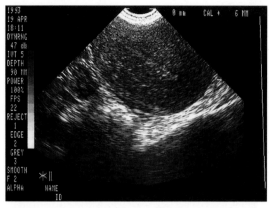

Figure 1 Postmenopausal uterus visualized by transvaginal ultrasound. Endometrial thickness was 6 mm. The patient was on continuous HRT for 7 years, with no vaginal bleeding

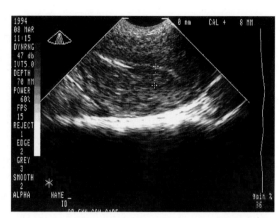

Figure 2 Endometrial thickness in a 58-year-old woman currently on sequential HRT for 2 years

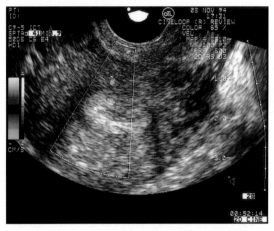

Figure 3 Transvaginal color Doppler was used to visualize endometrial blood flow in a postmenopausal woman with thickened endometrium. She was on HRT for 4 years, with occasional vaginal spotting

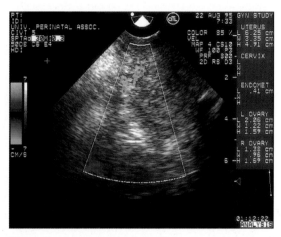

Figure 4 Another example of the postmenopausal uterus. Endometrial thickness was 41 mm and color Doppler was used to visualize intrauterine blood flow. The patient was a 61-year-old woman and she was on HRT for 11 years

best of our knowledge, as a contrast to the endometrium, myometrial thickness has not been extensively studied in postmenopausal women and under HRT. Our study attempted to establish the influence of age and HRT on myometrial thickness. None of these parameters showed profound increase or decrease in myometrial thickness.

The aging process also affected the uterine artery blood flow, but much less than we expected. The resistance to blood flow did not change significantly. Visualization of the uterine arteries decreased in both groups. Blood flow in the left and right uterine artery was approximately the same. Contrary to some previous publications, we did not observe that hormonal therapy changed uterine blood flow to a significant level. Bourne and colleagues[24] described the influence of transdermal estrogen and sequential oral norethisterone acetate on endometrial thickness and uterine artery blood flow after 6 weeks of HRT. They found a significant increase in endometrial thickness and decrease in blood flow impedance in ten postmenopausal

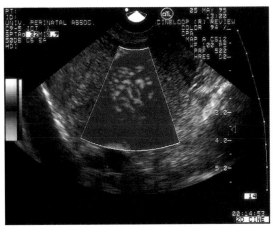

Figure 5 Power Doppler seems far superior to color Doppler in visualization of the small intrauterine vessels. Abundant blood supply on the myometrial–endometrial border in a 49-year-old patient. She was on HRT for only 1 year

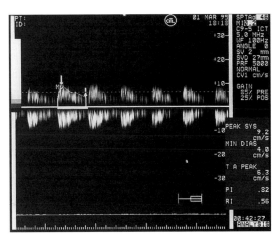

Figure 6 Pulsed Doppler waveform analysis of one small endometrial vessel in a 56-year-old woman. She had received HRT for 6 years

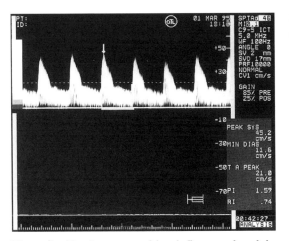

Figure 7 Uterine artery blood flow analyzed by pulsed Doppler in a postmenopausal woman receiving continuous HRT

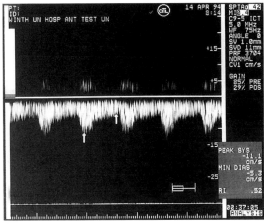

Figure 8 Another example of the intrauterine blood flow analyzed by pulsed Doppler in a patient on HRT for 3 years

women on HRT. All results were compared in patients before and after at least 6 weeks of therapy. The changes were profound (a 50% reduction in the pulsatility index) and occurred rapidly (within 6–10 weeks) when estrogens were administered non-orally. The other study from the same institution confirmed previous results with the conclusion that gonadal hormones have a profound effect on arterial tone in postmenopausal women[25]. This action may help explain some of the beneficial effects of

estrogen on arterial disease risk. Pines and colleagues[26] studied long-term effects of HRT on Doppler-derived parameters of aortic flow in postmenopausal women. Their results are more consistent with ours. The conclusion from the study was that the peripheral hemodynamic effects of HRT, such as vasodilatation, are transient, whereas the central effects (increased inotropism) are long lasting. More studies are required to clarify the present controversy on the influence of HRT on peripheral resistance.

Attention should be paid to the therapy protocol (unopposed estrogen, sequential regimens and continuous combined estrogen/progesterone regimens), the way of hormonal application (systemic or local), duration of therapy (months or years) and short- and long-term effects. The central and peripheral blood flow effects might not necessarily be the same.

RECENT STUDIES

Ultrasound has been gaining significance recently as a diagnostic tool not only in obstetrics but also in general gynecology. Improvements of image resolution by transvaginal sonography allow the investigation of even delicate anatomical structures such as the endometrium. The benefits of new technologies such as color Doppler and three-dimensional sonography are currently being assessed. In the postmenopausal patient without hormonal substitution, endometrial carcinoma may be diagnosed by measuring endometrial thickness alone. In women with postmenopausal bleeding endometrial atrophy as the most common cause has been differentiated from endometrial cancer with a high success rate. Considering that more than 70% of diagnostic curettages reveal benign pathology, sonography may significantly reduce the number of these procedures. In patients receiving HRT the measurement of endometrial thickness is not reliable, because the endometrium is subject to cyclical changes. Advantageous in this situation is the examination of the endometrial/myometrial border or endometrial blood flow. The potential of sonography in reducing the number of curettages has to be assessed in larger-scale prospective studies.

Pirhonen and co-workers[27] studied the effects of postmenopausal hormone replacement therapy on the uterus and uterine circulation. The study population consisted of 432 women of 58–59 years of age. Color Doppler ultrasonography with a transvaginal probe was used to measure the size of the uterus and the uterine artery pulsatility index. The mean endometrial thickness in group 1 (controls without HRT) was significantly thinner compared with group 2 (with HRT) and group 3 (after discontinuation of HRT). The mean uterine artery pulsatility index was lower in both groups 2 and 3 than in group 1. When HRT was initiated 2–10 years after menopause, the endometrial thickness did not differ from that among those who had started HRT earlier, but the pulsatility index was significantly higher. There was positive correlation between the size of the uterus and the pulsatility index in group 1, but the correlation was negative in group 2. In general, the duration of HRT had no effect on the pulsatility index. Estrogen users had a significantly thicker endometrium compared with estrogen–progestogen users. The pulsatility index was highest in the estrogen users with progestogen added every month. The authors concluded that the duration, onset of treatment in relation to menopause, discontinuation of HRT and mode of treatment modified both the normal postmenopausal endometrial thickness and the uterine vascular resistance.

Battaglia and colleagues[28] recently published a study aimed to compare the uterine blood flow variations induced by chemical castration and spontaneous menopause. Thirty infertile patients were studied in the early follicular phase (days 5–7) and then treated with gonadotropin releasing hormone agonists (GnRH-a). On day 25 from GnRH-a injection, the suppressive effect was checked. The values obtained were compared with those found in 18 postmenopausal women (menopause < 5 years). All the subjects underwent transvaginal ultrasonography, Doppler analysis of uterine arteries, hormonal assay and evaluation of hematological and biochemical parameters. In all infertile patients, the GnRH-a suppressive effect was shown at the 25th day from the injection. Endometrial thickness decreased from 0.6 ± 0.1 mm to 0.3 ± 0.1 mm ($p < 0.05$) and the pulsatility index increased from 2.52 ± 0.31 to 3.02 ± 0.25 ($p < 0.05$). The plasma estradiol level fell from 48.2 ± 4.4 pg/ml to 13.6 ± 7.9 pg/ml ($p < 0.05$). No other hormonal and biochemical parameters were significantly modified by GnRH-a. In postmenopausal women, the values of the studied parameters were similar to those found in the infertile GnRH-a-suppressed patients. These data show that GnRH-a induces vascular modifications similar to those induced soon after menopause and that both are probably exclusively related to hypoestrogenism.

Bonilla-Musoles and co-workers[29] used transvaginal color Doppler sonography to study the effect of hormone replacement on the uterine arterial blood flow of 203 postmenopausal women. The regimens studied involved estrogen replacement alone, continuous combined estrogen and progestogen, and estrogen followed sequentially by combined estrogen–progestogen. The mean pulsatility index fell to 0.65 ± 0.9 and the mean resistance index fell to 0.87 ± 0.4 during the first month of therapy ($p < 0.0001$). The addition of a progestogen did not alter the effect of estrogen alone ($p > 0.5$). Their findings suggest that the increase in vascular flow occurs even in women who begin therapy long after menopause. Contrary to this study, the same authors used transvaginal color Doppler sonography to study uterine artery blood flow velocity waveforms in 345 normal postmenopausal women who had never been on HRT[30]. Their objective was to establish the standard baseline flow values for normal postmenopausal women. The mean pulsatility index was 3.38 ± 1.04 and the mean resistance index was 0.93 ± 0.09. There was a positive correlation between arterial blood flow impedance and number of years since menopause. The authors believe that these levels may become important screening parameters for the detection of endometrial carcinoma in postmenopausal women.

An interesting issue is tamoxifen therapy. In menopausal patients with breast cancer who receive tamoxifen therapy, transvaginal sonography may show an abnormal endometrium. Achiron and associates[31] aimed to evaluate the effects of prolonged tamoxifen therapy on endometrial blood flow in postmenopausal patients with breast cancer, and to correlate blood flow characteristics with the sonographic appearance of the endometrium and its pathology. Transvaginal color Doppler ultrasound examinations were performed on 45 postmenopausal women (age range 54–70 years) with breast cancer, who had been treated with tamoxifen for 1–3 years. Twenty women (group

1) had a thick, irregular, cystic endometrium of ≥ 5 mm, and 25 (group 2) showed a thin endometrium of < 5 mm. The blood flow response was assessed by visualization of arterial waveforms in the endometrial and subendometrial regions with a transvaginal color flow imaging system. Resistance indexes were calculated for analysis and correlated with endometrial appearance and histology. The mean resistance index in group 1 was 0.39 ± 0.10 (range 0.32–0.54), and the mean resistance index in group 2 was 0.79 ± 0.10 (range 0.54–0.90; $p < 0.001$). On histology, 12 patients in group 1 showed atrophic endometrium confirmed by hysteroscopy, and in the remaining eight, endometrial polyps were found. In group 2, all patients had scanty, atrophic endometrium. Six of the eight patients with endometrial polyps had a resistance index of < 0.4 and none had malignant changes. These data suggest that tamoxifen therapy in women with postmenopausal breast cancer induces endometrial, morphological and blood flow changes, mimicking endometrial neoplasia.

In order to achieve non-invasive evaluation of the role of levonorgestrel-releasing devices in direct contact with the endometrium on menstrual spotting and endometrium inactivation, Pakarinen and colleagues[32] inserted levonorgestrel-releasing devices ($20\,\mu g/24\,h$) into either the cervical canal or the uterine cavity of 30 fertile women. Both before insertion and over the following 3 months, they used transvaginal sonography to measure the endometrial thickness in 20 of the women and Doppler flow to measure the uterine blood flow in the remaining ten women. The women were asked to keep records of menstrual bleeding and they gave blood samples for the measurement of serum estradiol, progesterone and levonorgestrel. By 10 weeks after insertion there was a significant decrease in endometrial thickness in both groups. Intracervical levonorgestrel release allowed the endometrium to maintain cyclic changes, whereas direct intrauterine levonorgestrel release eliminated the cyclical changes. The total number of spotting days was significantly less ($p = 0.0249$) in the intracervical release group at 3 months: 1.2 ± 0.6 vs. 8.1 ± 1.8

(mean ± SE). There were no significant differences in hormone concentrations between the groups. The pulsatility index did not change significantly during the study. The authors concluded that the inactivation process of the endometrium can be monitored by transvaginal sonography and that locally administered levonorgestrel does not produce circulatory changes detectable by Doppler flow. These results also suggest that the inactivation process of the endometrium is different between intracervical and intrauterine levonorgestrel administration and may explain the difference in the number of spotting days.

Handa and co-workers[33] wanted to test the hypothesis that a very-low-dose regimen of vaginal estrogen would provide effective relief from atrophic vaginitis without endometrial proliferation. Twenty postmenopausal women with symptoms, signs and cytological evidence of atrophic vaginitis were enrolled. Each subject was treated with 0.3 mg of conjugated estrogens, administered vaginally three nights per week for 6 months. They examined the following outcomes: symptoms, vaginal cellular (cytological) maturity, endometrial histology, sonographic evaluation of endometrial thickness, Doppler measures of uterine artery blood flow and serum levels of estrone and estradiol. Pre- and post-treatment data were compared for each subject. Satisfactory relief of symptoms occurred in 19 of 20 cases. Vaginal cellular maturation improved significantly with therapy ($p < 0.01$). There were no significant changes in endometrial thickness, uterine artery blood flow, or serum estrogen levels. Endometrial proliferation was observed in one case. The authors concluded that the relief from atrophic vaginitis can be achieved with 0.3 mg of conjugated estrogens administered vaginally three times per week. Endometrial proliferation may occur at this low dose, albeit rarely.

Kurjak and Kupesic[34] studied the flow velocity of the ovarian, uterine, radial and spiral arteries in different age groups. Serial measurements throughout the menstrual cycle in normally cycling women with documented fertility were compared with those in postmenopausal patients with and without HRT. A total of 250 patients were analyzed: 120 healthy fertile women, 85 postmenopausal patients and 45 postmenopausal patients receiving HRT. All patients were examined by transvaginal color and pulsed Doppler for changes in the resistance index of flow velocity waveforms of the ovarian, uterine radial and spiral arteries. Ovarian artery Doppler measurements in postmenopausal patients showed a significant difference when compared with the ovarian artery on the side containing a dominant follicle or corpus luteum in the healthy fertile group. Uterine and radial artery flow velocity analyses demonstrated significant positive correlation between the resistance index and years of menopause. In patients receiving HRT, a lowering effect occurred in the resistance index of the main uterine artery and its intramyometrial branches. Visualization of clear Doppler signals from the spiral arteries was possible in 30% of women who were menopausal for < 5 years. Increased vascular impedance was the typical finding in this vessel for this group of patients. The addition of HRT resulted in higher visualization rates of the spiral arteries and lowered resistance index values. The authors concluded that there are changes in the flow velocity patterns of the ovarian, uterine, radial and spiral arteries with age. The fact that the uterine artery resistance index does not change significantly in the first postmenopausal years strongly supports the thesis that the ageing process initially affects the uterus less than the ovary. Furthermore, the uterine environment can be manipulated more easily during the menopausal years by proper hormonal stimulation.

Achiron and colleagues[35] evaluated the endometrial blood flow response to hormone replacement therapy in women with premature ovarian failure who planned to enter an oocyte donation program. Transvaginal color Doppler ultrasound examinations were performed in women with ovarian failure before and during a cycle of standard HRT and in those with normal menstrual cycles. Blood flow response was assessed by visualization of arterial waveforms in the endometrial region. The transvaginal color flow imaging system was used. Resistance indexes were calculated for analysis and correlated with plasma estradiol and progesterone concentrations for 18 women with ovarian failure (study group) and 12 volunteers with normal ovarian cycles (control group). Data for resistance indexes were divided into five phases according to the day of hormonal cycle: 0, pretreatment phase; I, early follicular phase (days 5–7); II, late follicular phase (days 11–13); III, early luteal phase (days 17–21); and IV, late luteal phase (days 23–25). All women with ovarian failure demonstrated continuous forward end-diastolic flow velocities at phase I, whereas none showed this pattern during the pretreatment period (phase 0). Women with ovarian failure in the early follicular phase had a significantly higher resistance index (0.85 ± 0.1; mean $\pm$ SD) than that in the late follicular phase (0.57 ± 0.1), and the resistance index in the early luteal phase (0.67 ± 0.1) was significantly higher than that of the late follicular phase. There was no difference in the resistance index between early and late luteal phases. A similar pattern of lower resistance index around midcycle was observed in the control group. However, a comparison of the resistance indexes between patients with ovarian failure and control patients revealed a significant difference between values in the early follicular phase only (0 ± 0.1 vs. 0.68 ± 0.1). In the late follicular phase and during the entire luteal phase, the mean resistance index did not differ between the study and control groups. The authors concluded that standard HRT in women with premature ovarian failure enables restoration of endometrial blood flow to normal. This may imply uterine receptivity for oocyte donation.

Pines and colleagues[26] studied the long-term effects of HRT on Doppler-derived parameters of aortic flow in postmenopausal women. Eighteen postmenopausal women were examined by Doppler echocardiography before initiation of HRT (T1), then after 10 weeks (T2) and 1 year (T3). This study group was compared with another in which HRT was not used. Flow velocity integral, and an indicator of cardiac contractility were calculated. In the study group, PFV was 107 ± 18 cm/s at T1 and increased significantly at T2 and T3. Ejection time, which was prolonged at T2 compared to T1, returned to its basal value at T3. The flow velocity integral increased at T2, but this change was only partially sustained at T3. Mean acceleration maintained its increase throughout T2 to T3. None of the Doppler parameters showed a significant change in the controls from T1 to T3. Their our results suggest that the peripheral hemodynamic effects of HRT, such as vasodilatation, are transient, whereas the central effects (increased inotropism) are long-lasting.

Cardiovascular risk is higher in men than in women, and also more prevalent in postmenopausal than in premenopausal women, especially if not treated by estrogens. These differences may be due, in part, to a cardioprotective action of sex hormones, mainly estrogens. However, only a limited part of this protection may be attributed to metabolic modifications induced by replacement therapy with estrogen. Therefore, it remains to be determined which other cardioprotective mechanisms influenced by sex steroids might be involved. It has been demonstrated that the menopause is associated with an increase in uterine arterial pulsatility index, reflecting increased peripheral resistance, whereas the administration of estrogens has an opposite effect at this level. In Doppler studies, estrogen replacement therapy was also associated with an increase in stroke volume and flow acceleration in the aorta. This suggests a positive inotropic effect of estrogens. With the use of technetium scanning, it was found that women at an early phase of menopause had a stronger myocardial contractility than women of a similar age whose menopause was of longer duration. These effects of estrogens on hemodynamic characteristics might be controlled by vasoregulatory hormones such as endothelin(s) or endothelial-derived relaxing factor, now identified as nitric oxide. Indeed, associated differences in endothelin have been observed. At present, conclusive data are not available.

CONCLUSIONS

Hormonal replacement therapy offers significant benefits to many postmenopausal women, especially to those whose menopause occurred before age 45. In addition, women at high risk for atherosclerosis or who already have cardiovascular disease would particularly benefit from estrogen use. The increased risk of endometrial and breast cancer seen with estrogen replacement appears to be small in comparison with its protective effect against cardiovascular disease. The benefits and risks as they pertain to each individual patient should be reviewed with her in detail. Transvaginal ultrasound and Doppler blood flow analysis might prove helpful in management of patients on HRT to prevent unwanted effects. Ultimately, the patient must decide whether or not to initiate therapy and give her informed consent.

References

1. Henderson, B. E., Paganini-Hill, A. and Ross, R. K. (1991). Decreased mortality in users of estrogen replacement therapy. *Arch. Intern. Med.*, **151**, 75–8

2. Stampfer, M. J., Willett, W. C., Colditz, G. A., Rosner, B., Speizer, F. E. and Hennekens, C. H. (1985). A prospective study of postmenopausal estrogen therapy and coronary heart disease. *N. Engl. J. Med.*, **313**, 1044–9

3. Hunt, K., Vessey, M., McPherson, K. and Coleman, M. (1987). Long-term surveillance of mortality and cancer incidence in women receiving hormone replacement therapy. *Br. J. Obstet. Gynaecol.*, **94**, 620–35

4. WHO Scientific Group (1981). Research on the menopause. *World Health Organ. Tech. Rep. Ser.*, **670**, 53–68

5. Antunes, C. M., Strolley, P. D., Rosenshein, N. B. *et al.* (1979). Endometrial cancer and estrogen use: report of a large case–control study. *N. Engl. J. Med.*, **300**, 9–13

6. Chu, J., Scweid, A. I. and Weiss, N. S. (1982). Survival among women with endometrial cancer: a comparison of estrogen users and non-users. *Am. J. Obstet. Gynecol.*, **143**, 569–73

7. Shapiro, S., Kelly, J. P., Rosenberg, L. *et al.* (1985). Risk of localized and widespread endometrial cancer in relation to recent and discontinued use of conjugated estrogen. *N. Engl. J. Med.*, **313**, 969–72

8. Rubin, G. L., Peterson, H. B., Lee, N. C., Maes, E. F., Wingo, P. A. and Becker, S. (1990). Estrogen replacement therapy and the risk of endometrial cancer; remaining controversies. *Am. J. Obstet. Gynecol.*, **162**, 148–54

9. Steinberg, K. K., Thacker, S. B., Smith, S. J., Stroup, D. F., Zack, M. M., Flanders, W. D. and Berkleman, R. L. (1991). A meta-analysis of the effect of estrogen replacement therapy on the risk of breast cancer. *J. Am. Med. Assoc.*, **265**, 1985–90

10. Nasri, M. N. B., Shepherd, J. H., Setchell, M. E. *et al.* (1991). The role of vaginal scan in measurement of endometrial thickness in postmenopausal women. *Br. J. Obstet. Gynaecol.*, **98**, 470–5

11. Wikland, M., Granberg, S. and Karlsson, B. (1992). Assessment of the endometrium in the postmenopausal woman by vaginal ultrasound. *Ultrasound Q.*, **10**, 15–27

12. Barber, H. R. K. (1988). *Perimenopausal and Geriatric Gynecology*, pp. 207–17. (New York: Macmillan)

13. Gambrell, R. D. (1982). The menopause: benefits and risk of estrogen–progesterone replacement therapy. *Fertil. Steril.*, **37**, 457–61

14. Varner, R. E. (1990). Hormone replacement therapy. In Shingleton, H. M. and Hurt, W. G. (eds.) *Reproductive Gynecology*, pp. 143–69. (New York: Churchill Livingstone)

15. Gibbons, W. E., Moyer, D. L., Lobo, R. A. *et al.* (1986). Biochemical and histologic effects on sequential estrogen/progestin therapy on the endometrium of postmenopausal women. *Am. J. Obstet. Gynecol.*, **154**, 456–9

16. Prough, S., Aksel, S., Wieb, R. *et al.* (1987). Continuous estrogen/progestin therapy in menopause. *Am. J. Obstet. Gynecol.*, **157**, 1449–52

17. Kurjak, A. and Zalud, I. (1991). Uterine masses. In Kurjak, A. (ed.) *Transvaginal Color Doppler*, pp.123–35. (Carnforth, UK: Parthenon Publishing)

18. Fleischer, A. C., Gordon, A. N., Entman, S. S. *et al.* (1990). Transvaginal scanning of the endometrium. *J. Clin. Ultrasound*, **18**, 337–41

19. Jones, H. W. III (1988). Cyclic histology and cytology of the genital tract. In Jones, H. W. III, Wentz, A. C. and Burnett, L. S. (eds.) *Novak's Textbook of Gynecology*, pp. 68–88. (Baltimore: Williams and Wilkins)

20. Sadan, O., van Iddekinge, B., Savange, N. *et al.* (1990). Endocrine profile associated with estrogen and progesterone receptors in leiomyoma

and normal myometrium. *Gynecol. Endocrinol.*, **4**, 33–7

21. Fleischer, A. C., Kepple, D. M. and Entman, S. S. (1991). Transvaginal sonography of uterine disorders. In Timor-Tritsch, I. E. and Rottem, S. (eds.) *Transvaginal Sonography*, pp. 109–30. (New York: Elsevier)

22. Zalud, I., Conway, C., Schulman, H. and Trinca, D. (1993). Endometrial and myometrial thickness and uterine blood flow in postmenopausal women: the influence of hormonal replacement therapy and age. *J. Ultrasound Med.*, **12**, 737–41

23. Varner, R. E., Sparks, J. M., Cameron, C. D., Roberts, L. L. and Soong, S. J. (1991). Transvaginal sonography of the endometrium in postmenopausal women. *Obstet. Gynecol.*, **78**, 195–9

24. Bourne, T., Hillard, T. C., Whitehead, M. I., Crook, D. and Campbell, S. (1990). Oestrogens, arterial status, and postmenopausal women (letter). *Lancet*, **335**, 1470–1

25. Hillard, T. C., Bourne, T. H., Whitehead, M. I., Crayford, T. B., Collins, W. P. and Campbell, S. (1992). Differential effects of transdermal estradiol and sequential progesterone on impedance to flow within the uterine arteries of postmenopausal women. *Fertil. Steril.*, **58**, 959–63

26. Pines, A., Fisman, E. Z., Aylon, D., Drory, Y., Averbuch, M. and Levro, Y. (1992). Long-term effects of hormone replacement therapy on Doppler-derived parameters of aortic flow in postmenopausal women. *Chest*, **102**, 1496–8

27. Pirhonen, J. R., Vuento, M. H., Makinen, J. I. and Salmi, T. A. (1993). Long-term effects of hormone replacement therapy on the uterus and on uterine circulation. *Am. J. Obstet. Gynecol.*, **168**, 620–30

28. Battaglia, C., Artini, P. G., Bencini, S., Bianchi, R., D'Ambrogio, G. and Genazzani, A. R. (1995). Doppler analysis of uterine blood flow changes in spontaneous and medically induced menopause. *Gynecol. Endocrinol.*, **9**, 143–8

29. Bonilla-Musoles, F., Marti, M. C., Ballester, M. J., Raga, F. and Osborne, N. G. (1995). Normal uterine arterial blood flow in postmenopausal women assessed by transvaginal color Doppler sonography: the effect of hormone replacement therapy. *J. Ultrasound Med.*, **14**, 497–501

30. Bonilla-Musoles, F., Marti, M. C., Ballester, M. J., Raga, F. and Osborne, N. G. (1995). Normal uterine arterial blood flow in postmenopausal women assessed by transvaginal color Doppler ultrasonography. *J. Ultrasound Med.*, **14**, 491–4

31. Achiron, R., Lipitz, S., Sivan, E., Goldenberg, M., Horovitz, A., Frenkel, Y. and Mashiach, S. (1995). Changes mimicking endometrial neoplasia in postmenopausal, tamoxifen-treated women with breast cancer: a transvaginal Doppler study. *Ultrasound Obstet. Gynecol.*, **6**, 116–20

32. Pakarinen, P., Luukkainen, T., Lame, H. and Lahteenmaki, P. (1995). The effect of local intrauterine levongestrel administration on endometrial thickness and uterine blood circulation. *Hum. Reprod.*, **10**, 2390–4

33. Handa, V. L., Bachus, K. E., Johnston, W. W., Robboy, S. J. and Hammond, C. B. (1994). Vaginal administration of low-dose conjugated estrogen: systemic absorption and effects on the endometrium. *Obstet. Gynecol.*, **84**, 215–18

34. Kurjak, A. and Kupesic, S. (1995). Ovarian senescence and its significance on uterine and ovarian perfusion. *Fertil. Steril.*, **64**, 532–7

35. Achiron, H., Levran, D., Sivan, E., Lipitz, S., Dor, J. and Mashiach, S. (1995). Endometrial blood flow response to hormone replacement therapy in women with premature ovarian failure: a transvaginal Doppler study. *Fertil. Steril.*, **63**, 550–4

Reproducibility of gynecological Doppler measurements

14

L. Valentin

INTRODUCTION

With the introduction of color Doppler it became possible to assess blood flow velocities in very small parenchymal vessels. This new technique has been used for the assessment of physiological changes in the blood circulation of the uterus and ovaries[1–4], for the evaluation of infertility[5–9] and for the differentiation of benign and malignant adnexal tumors[10–12]. However, there are problems with regard to the application of these techniques. One crucial problem is the intra- and interobserver variability in Doppler measurements of blood flow velocity. The reliability of Doppler measurements has been questioned, even where relatively large and well defined vessels such as the umbilical artery, the fetal aorta and the fetal internal carotid artery are concerned[13]. Despite the importance of the reproducibility issue in general, little has been published on the reproducibility of Doppler measurements in gynecological applications.

HOW SHOULD REPRODUCIBILITY BE MEASURED?

The optimal statistical approach to the assessment of intra- and interobserver reproducibility is not obvious. The product-moment correlation coefficient (r) between the results of repeated measurements has been used as an indicator of agreement in some studies, such as that by Serfontein and Jaroszewies[14]. However, strong correlation does not mean that two values agree, but only that they are related[15], which they ought to be as they represent measurements of the same thing. In other studies, the coefficient of variation has been used as the sole measure of reproducibility[9,16–21]. It is probably incorrect to use the coefficient of variation alone to assess the reliability of repeated measurements, as even a high error variance may be compatible with a low coefficient of variation[13]. Alternative analyses of reproducibility (agreement between measurements made by two different observers or repeatability of measurements made by one observer) have been described by Bland and Altman[15,22], Brennan and Silman[23], Burdock and co-workers[24], Kramer and Feinstein[25], Scherjon and colleagues[13] and Cohen[26].

When assessing interobserver reproducibility (i.e. agreement between measurements made by two independent observers) of continuous data, one might start by plotting the differences between corresponding measurements against the respective means of the two sets of data. Such a plot provides an overview of the magnitude of differences between the two sets of measurements and allows investigation of a possible relationship between the 'measurement error' (i.e. the difference between the two sets of data) and the 'true value' (i.e. the mean of the two sets of data, which is the best available estimate of 'truth'). If there is no obvious relationship between the difference and the mean, we can summarize the lack of agreement between the two observers by calculating the mean difference (d) and the standard deviation of the differences (s). If the differences are normally distributed (which they usually are), 95% of the differences will lie between $d - 1.96s$ and $d + 1.96s$. These limits are called the limits of agreement[15]. The precision of the estimated mean difference and limits of agreement can be determined by calculating the 95% confidence intervals for the mean difference and lower and upper limits of agreement[15]. If the 95% confidence interval for the mean interobserver difference brackets zero, no systematic bias exists between the two observers, i.e. there is no reason to believe that one observer consistently obtains higher or lower values than the other[23]. If, on the other hand, the 95% confidence interval does not bracket zero, there is a systematic difference between the two observers. In some cases, the plot will show the difference to be related to the mean, the difference often increasing with the mean. Logarithmic transformation may eliminate or reduce such a relationship. If so, the analysis described above can be applied to the log-transformed data. The antilogs of the mean difference and of the limits of agreement calculated from the log-transformed data yield the results in terms of a ratio. If the antilogs of the lower and upper limits of agreement are 0.80 and 1.20, respectively, this means that in 95% of cases observer 2 will obtain measurements which are between 0.80 and 1.20 times those of observer 1[15,23], i.e. measurements which are between 80% and 120% of those of observer 1. How far apart measurements made by two different observers can be without causing problems is a clinical judgement.

Provided that only two repeated measurements are performed, an approach similar to that outlined above can be used to calculate intraobserver reproducibility (i.e. the repeatability of measurements made by the same observer) of continuous data. If there are more than two repeated measurements the calculations are more complex and include the use of one-way analysis of variance[15]. In the latter case, the 'measurement error' can be expressed as the within-subject standard deviation (i.e. the square root of the within-subject mean square error). The coefficient of variation can be calculated as the quotient of the within-subject standard deviation divided by the mean of all recorded values, expressed as a percentage.

Another way of measuring inter- and intraobserver reproducibility is to calculate the inter- and intraclass correlation coefficients[13,22,24,25]. Inter- and intraclass correlation coefficients indicate the proportion of the total variance in measurement results which can be explained by differences between the individuals examined, a high inter- or intraclass correlation coefficient indicating that the measurements can be used to discriminate between individuals. As a rule, values for inter- and intraclass correlation coefficients above 0.75 are said to be acceptable[24], although the use of so strict a cut-off level has been criticized[22]. In one sense, inter- and intraclass correlation coefficients may be thought of as representing the degree to which repeated measurements contain the same information[22]. However, as inter- and intraclass correlation coefficients are dependent on the variance in the population, they are insufficient to assess whether a measurement method yields consistent results. If the population variance is high, high values will be obtained for inter- and intraclass correlation coefficients, especially if the within-subject variance is low; the more variable the subjects, the greater the inter- and intraclass correlation coefficients, and the less variable the subjects the smaller the inter- and intraclass correlation coefficients. Thus, inter- and intraclass correlation coefficients are applicable only to a particular population. Therefore, when agreement or repeatability is assessed, not only should inter- and intraclass correlation coefficients be taken into account, but also 'measurement errors' in absolute terms (e.g. mean difference, limits of agreement, within-subject standard deviation or coefficient of variation).

Cohen's Kappa can be used to assess inter- and intraobserver agreement for categorical data[23,26]. Cohen's Kappa is the ratio of the observed accuracy beyond chance to the maximum achievable accuracy beyond chance [Kappa = $(P_o - P_e)/(1 - P_e)$, where P_o is the observed proportion of individuals tested where the two measurements agree, and P_e is the proportion of individuals where the two measurements could be expected to agree on the basis of chance alone]. Cohen's Kappa has a maximum value of +1, values of 0.81–1.0 indicating excellent agreement between results, values of 0.61–0.80 good agreement and values of 0.41–0.60 moderate agreement[23].

DETERMINANTS OF WITHIN-SUBJECT VARIANCE IN GYNECOLOGICAL DOPPLER MEASUREMENTS

Differences in sample site probably explain much of the within-subject variance in gynecological Doppler measurements. Imagine two observers given the task of obtaining the highest possible Doppler shift from an artery in the ovarian stroma, in the wall of the dominant follicle or corpus luteum, or in a tumor. Because many arteries are detectable at color Doppler ultrasound examination of these structures, it is very unlikely that the two observers will sample exactly the same artery at exactly the same site – if they perform their examinations independently of each other. A single observer, too, would almost certainly have difficulty in relocating a previous sample site in an ovary or tumor if he/she were to repeat each examination from the very beginning. It may be difficult to relocate exactly a previous sample site, even in the large and well-defined uterine artery, the reason being the extreme tortuousness of this vessel with several vessel loops detectable at the recommended sample site 'lateral to the cervix at the level of the internal os'. One would expect the reproducibility of Doppler measurements to improve, if the Doppler gate were not to be moved between repeated measurements. However, such 'fixed sample site' reproducibility studies would not be very interesting from a clinical point of view, because what we really want to know is whether the same observer or two different observers can arrive at the same result when a Doppler examination is performed from the very beginning – including the selection of the most appropriate sample site.

Another source of error is the dependence of Doppler velocimetry results on the insonation angle. However, owing to the small and tortuous nature of the vessels examined, correction for the angle of insonation is usually impossible in gynecological ultrasonography. Moreover, angle correction is possible only vis-à-vis the scanning plane; and as the vessel examined may be misaligned with the scanning plane, a component of the angle between flow direction and scanning plane might go uncorrected for. Even if the highest possible Doppler shifts from each vessel examined are sought, blood flow velocity cannot be precisely measured in that way. On the other hand, because the blood flow velocity waveform index is a ratio between velocities, its value is little affected by the insonation angle, provided that blood flow velocities are recorded throughout diastole.

A third source of error when performing Doppler measurements is the variation in results introduced by the analysis of the Doppler shift spectrum. A study that assesses only the reproducibility of the analysis of preselected spectra will show much less within-subject variance than a study that assesses the reproducibility of the entire examination procedure including the selection of representative spectra.

If a reproducibility study extends over some time, physiological changes occurring during the examination may account for a considerable proportion of the within-subject variance in Doppler results. Heart rate is one physiological factor that may affect the blood flow velocity waveform. Maternal heart rate has been shown to affect the arcuate artery pulsatility index in pregnant women[27], and fetal heart rate to affect the blood flow velocity waveform index in the umbilical artery and descending fetal aorta[28–31]. On the other hand, the ultrasound examiner has the possibility of controlling for this factor by trying to obtain Doppler shift spectra with approximately the same heart rate. Simultaneous intrauterine pressure recordings and transvaginal Doppler measurements have shown uterine contractions to exert marked effects on uterine artery blood flow velocity waveforms (Valentin, Sladkevicius and Marsàl, unpublished data). The uterus contracts in both pre- and postmenopausal women, and the uterine contractility pattern changes during the menstrual cycle[32,33]. Unless intrauterine pressure recordings are performed simultaneously with the Doppler ultrasound examination, this physiological factor cannot be controlled for by the examiner. Other physiological changes affecting the blood flow velocity waveforms in uterine or ovarian arteries – but beyond the control of the ultrasound examiner – may occur as well.

Other sources of within-subject variance are observer bias, interaction between observer and subject, and unspecified variability (e.g. distracting elements in an observational setting).

HOW SHOULD A REPRODUCIBILITY STUDY BE DESIGNED?

From the foregoing it is obvious that the results of a reproducibility study will be highly dependent on its design. A study which examines only the reproducibility of the analysis of preselected Doppler shift spectra will show less within-subject variance (i.e. 'better' results) than such a study designed to determine the reproducibility of the selection of representative spectra as well. A study using a 'fixed sample site' will almost certainly show less within-subject variance than a study in which the sample site has to be relocated before each new measurement. A reproducibility study with a very short observation period will probably show less within-subject variance than a study extending over a longer observation period, when there is greater risk of physiological changes that will affect the results. Other factors which probably affect the results of reproducibility studies of Doppler measurements are the number of repeated measurements performed, the number of heartbeats analyzed and the method of analyzing the spectra (e.g. on-line or off-line analysis).

The ideal design of a reproducibility study is not intuitively apparent. From one point of view, a short observation period might seem desirable to minimize the effect of physiological changes on the results, the argument for this being that, after all, a reproducibility study should determine only 'measurement errors' and not physiological changes. On the other hand, uncontrollable physiological changes (such as the effect of uterine contractions on uterine artery Doppler shift spectra) might render a Doppler ultrasound examination clinically useless, and thus a longer observation period taking such changes into account might seem more appropriate. The ideal Doppler reproducibility study would seem to be one with an observation period short enough to exclude the effects of physiological variations but nonetheless taking

into account all sources of measurement error (finding the sample site, obtaining an optimal and representative spectrum and analyzing the spectrum), and where each new measurement is unbiased by previous measurements. Unfortunately, such a study would probably be practically unfeasible, at least if intraobserver reproducibility were to be measured, because if the observer is to be unbiased when repeating measurements, some time must elapse between the measurements to allow him/her to forget the previous ones (especially the exact sample site); thus a rather long observation period would probably be necessary.

At the very least, the study design and the methodology must be described in detail in every reproducibility study. Only then can the reader put the results into context and evaluate their clinical importance.

HOW REPRODUCIBLE ARE DOPPLER ULTRASOUND MEASUREMENTS OF BLOOD FLOW VELOCITIES IN THE UTERINE AND OVARIAN ARTERIES?

Several research teams have reported the reproducibility of Doppler measurements from the uterine and/or ovarian arteries to be good, coefficients of variation of approximately 10% being obtained in postmenopausal women[16] and of 4–11% in premenopausal women[9,17–21]. However, as the methods of collecting and analyzing the data were not described in these reports, it is impossible to evaluate the clinical importance of the results (see previous sections in this chapter).

To the best of my knowledge, the first report on the reproducibility of gynecological Doppler measurements to include an appropriate description of the study design was published in 1989 by Farquar and co-workers[34]. In that study, the transabdominal examination technique without the aid of color Doppler was used. The authors concluded that the reproducibility of Doppler measurements in the uterine and ovarian arteries was unsatisfactory, and that Doppler examinations of pelvic vessels in non-pregnant women were insufficiently reliable for research purposes.

Some reports of more recent reproducibility studies using the color Doppler technique as an aid in measuring blood flow velocities in the uterine and ovarian arteries have included at least a partial description of the study design and methodology[35-39]. The results are summarized in Tables 1–4. Ranges of values are given in some of the columns of the tables. This is because in some studies reproducibility was assessed separately for the left and right uterine arteries[35,36], separately for different sites in the ovary (hilum,

stroma, follicle, corpus luteum)[35] and separately for the follicular and luteal phases of the menstrual cycle[35]. In another study[37], different types of reproducibility were evaluated, i.e. 'beat-to-beat' reproducibility (for which two consecutive heart beats in the same frozen frame were analyzed), 'frame-to-frame' reproducibility (for which heart beats in different frames of the same cine loop were analyzed) and 'temporal' reproducibility (for which measurements were taken 15 min apart and included relocation of the

Table 1 Inter- and intraobserver reproducibility of Doppler measurements of uterine artery pulsatility index

Study	TAS or TVS	Pre- or post-MP	Interobserver reproducibility		Intraobserver reproducibility	
			CV (%)	Inter-CC	CV (%)	Intra-CC
Sladkevicius and Valentin[35]	TVS	pre-MP	9–21	0.61–0.88	14; 19	0.72; 0.36
Sladkevicius and Valentin[36]	TVS	post-MP	10; 14	0.89; 0.66	7; 14	0.96; 0.79
Steer et al.[38]	TVS	pre MP	12	—	4; 5	—
Steer et al.[38]	TAS	pre-MP	—	—	7; 11	—
Tekay and Jouppila[37]	TVS	pre-MP	—	—	6–12	0.96–0.99

TAS, transabdominal sonography; TVS, transvaginal sonography; pre-MP, premenopausal subjects; post-MP, postmenopausal subjects; CV, coefficient of variation; Inter-CC, interclass correlation coefficient; Intra-CC, intraclass correlation coefficient

Table 2 Inter- and intraobserver reproducibility of Doppler measurements of uterine artery time-averaged maximum velocity (TAMXV) and peak systolic velocity (PSV)

Study	TAS or TVS	Pre- or post-MP	TAMXV or PSV	Interobserver reproducibility		Intraobserver reproducibility	
				CV (%)	Inter-CC	CV (%)	Intra-CC
Sladkevicius and Valentin[35]	TVS	pre-MP	TAMXV	18–20	0.63–0.80	14; 24	0.78; 0.36
Sladkevicius and Valentin[36]	TVS	post-MP	TAMXV	22; 41	0.78; 0.53	18; 22	0.80; 0.85
Tekay and Jouppila[37]	TVS	pre-MP	PSV	—	—	1–15	0.88–0.99

TAS, transabdominal sonography; TVS, transvaginal sonography; pre-MP, premenopausal subjects; post-MP, postmenopausal subjects; CV, coefficient of variation; Inter-CC, interclass correlation coefficient; Intra-CC, intraclass correlation coefficient

Table 3 Inter- and intraobserver reproducibility of Doppler measurements of pulsatility index in intraovarian arteries

Study	TAS or TVS	Pre- or post-MP	Interobserver reproducibility		Intraobserver reproducibility	
			CV (%)	Inter-CC	CV (%)	Intra-CC
Sladkevicius and Valentin[35]	TVS	pre-MP	13–17	0.34–0.58	8–15	0.31–0.82
Sladkevicius and Valentin[36]	TVS	post-MP	22	0.31	—	—
Tekay and Jouppila[37]	TVS	pre-MP	—	—	9–19	0.78–0.95

TAS, transabdominal sonography; TVS, transvaginal sonography; pre-MP, premenopausal subjects; post-MP, postmenopausal subjects; CV, coefficient of variation; Inter-CC, interclass correlation coefficient; Intra-CC, intraclass correlation coefficient sample site). In the latter study, 'beat-to-beat' reproducibility and 'frame-to-frame' reproducibility were very good, whereas 'temporal' reproducibility was less satisfactory[37]. The differences in results between the studies listed in Tables 1–4 may well be explained by differences in study design and methodology. They do not necessarily reflect differences in the ability to obtain reproducible results.

Limits of agreement were calculated in three studies[35,36,39]. Even though the mean differences between repeated measurements were small, the ranges between the lower and upper

limits of agreement were very wide (Tables 5 and 6).

The results presented in Tables 1–6 indicate that uterine artery measurements are more reproducible than ovarian artery measurements, and that measurements of the pulsatility index are more reproducible than those of time-averaged maximum velocity and peak systolic velocity. It is not surprising that consistency in the results of Doppler measurements in the uterine arteries is better than that of measurements in the ovarian arteries, as the uterine artery is a well-defined vessel that can be

Table 4 Inter- and intraobserver reproducibility of Doppler measurements of time-averaged maximum velocity (TAMXV) and peak systolic velocity (PSV) in intraovarian arteries

Study	TAS or TVS	Pre- or post-MP	TAMXV or PSV	Interobserver reproducibility CV (%)	Inter-CC	Intraobserver reproducibility CV (%)	Intra-CC
Sladkevicius and Valentin[35]	TVS	pre-MP	TAMXV	22–34	0.10–0.76	29–39	0.16–0.69
Sladkevicius and Valentin[36]	TVS	post-MP	TAMXV	23	0.47	—	—
Tekay and Jouppila[37]	TVS	pre-MP	PSV	—	—	2–16	0.63–0.99

TAS, transabdominal sonography; TVS, transvaginal sonography; pre-MP, premenopausal subjects; post-MP, postmenopausal subjects; CV, coefficient of variation; Inter-CC, interclass correlation coefficient; Intra-CC, intraclass correlation coefficient

Table 5 Inter- and intraobserver reproducibility: mean difference and lower and upper limits of agreement for measurements of pulsatility index (PI) in uterine and intraovarian arteries

Measurement	Mean measurement value	Mean difference	Lower limit	Upper limit
Uterine artery PI, interobserver				
Post-MP, right[36]	2.3	−0.02	−0.98	0.94
Post-MP, left[36]	2.3	0.10	−0.59	0.79
Follicular phase, dom.[35]	2.4	0.13	−0.66	0.92
Follicular phase, non-dom.[35]	2.4	0.22	−1.36	1.81
Luteal phase, dom.[35]	2.5	0.13	−0.59	0.85
Luteal phase, non-dom.[35]	2.6	0.02	−0.78	0.82
Pre-MP, unknown cycle day[39]	—	0.05	−0.87	0.96
Uterine artery PI, intraobserver				
Pre-MP, unknown cycle day[39]	—	0.06	−0.91	1.03
Intraovarian artery PI, interobserver				
Post-MP[36]	1.1	0.11	−0.65	0.87
Dominant follicle[35]	0.7	0.02	−0.26	0.31
Corpus luteum[35]	0.6	−0.05	−0.27	0.17
Stroma non-dom., follicular phase[35]	0.8	−0.04	−0.40	0.32
Stroma non-dom., luteal phase[35]	0.7	−0.04	−0.49	0.40

Post-MP, postmenopausal subjects; Pre-MP, premenopausal subjects; dom., side harboring the dominant follicle or corpus luteum; non-dom., side contralateral to the dominant side

Table 6 Inter- and intraobserver reproducibility: mean difference and lower and upper limits of agreement for measurements of time-averaged maximum velocity (TAMXV) and in uterine and intraovarian arteries

Measurement	Mean measurement value (cm/s)	Mean difference (cm/s)	Lower limit (cm/s)	Upper limit (cm/s)
Uterine artery TAMXV, interobserver				
Post-MP, right[36]	13.5	−1.6	−17.9	14.6
Post-MP, left[36]	11.8	−1.2	−8.8	6.4
Follicular phase, dom.[35]	22.8	−2.3	−14.9	10.2
Follicular phase, non-dom.[35]	19.8	0.8	−10.7	12.3
Luteal phase, dom.[35]	20.9	−2.7	−13.5	8.1
Luteal phase, non-dom.[35]	19.1	0.4	−12.1	12.9
Intraovarian artery TAMXV, interobserver				
Post-MP[36]	2.4	−0.4	−1.9	1.2
Dominant follicle[35]	12.8	2.2	−11.1	15.6
Corpus luteum[35]	32.8	−2.5	−37.0	31.9
Stroma non-dom., follicular phase[35]	6.8	0.2	−5.3	5.7
Stroma non-dom., luteal phase[35]	10.6	0.7	−7.6	9.0

Post-MP, postmenopausal subjects; Pre-MP, premenopausal subjects; dom., side harboring the dominant follicle or corpus luteum; non-dom., side contralateral to the dominant side

sampled at a defined site (lateral to the cervix at the level of the internal os), whereas it is much more difficult (not to say impossible) to define a fixed sample site for intraovarian arteries. Like us[40], another research team[41] have found it very difficult to identify with certainty the main ovarian artery in the infundibulopelvic ligament. Thus, it is not a viable alternative to sample the main ovarian artery instead of intraovarian arteries. Given the angle dependency of velocity measurements, it was also to be expected that time-averaged maximum velocity and peak systolic velocity would be measured less reliably than the pulsatility index. The wide ranges between the lower and upper limits of agreement illustrate that it is very difficult to obtain reproducible results of Doppler measurements of blood flow velocities in uterine and intraovarian arteries in both pre- and postmenopausal women.

It may well be questioned whether the results of the reproducibility studies cited[35–39] can be generalized as valid for all Doppler examinations carried out with similar methodology, or whether the results are valid only for the observers involved in the respective studies. However, as these observers were experienced examiners, I venture to make the following generalizations: the results of studies in which the Doppler technique was used to investigate physiological changes in the blood circulation of the uterus and ovaries must be interpreted with caution; neither the intra- nor the interobserver reproducibility of Doppler measurements in intraovarian arteries seems to be good enough to allow the detection of small differences in the pulsatility index, time-averaged maximum velocity or peak systolic velocity; one can expect to detect only large differences; uterine artery Doppler measurements would seem to be more reliable, and it might well be possible to detect fairly small differences in the uterine artery pulsatility index; and finally, it is less likely that small differences in time-averaged maximum velocity could be detected in the uterine arteries.

HOW REPRODUCIBLE ARE RESULTS OF DOPPLER ULTRASOUND EXAMINATIONS OF GYNECOLOGICAL TUMORS?

To the best of my knowledge, only two reports have been published on the reproducibility of Doppler ultrasound examinations of gynecological tumors[42,43]. The first study was designed by Sladkevicius and myself to evaluate interobserver agreement in the results of Doppler measurements of peak systolic velocity,

Table 7 Inter-observer agreement in measurements of peak systolic velocity (PSV), time-averaged maximum velocity (TAMXV), pulsatility index (PI) and tumor color score in extrauterine pelvic tumors[42]

	Geometric mean of values measured	Mean difference (%)	Limits of agreement (%)		
			Lower	Upper	Inter-CC
Highest tumor PSV (cm/s)	22.1	−1	−73	235	0.67
Highest tumor TAMXV (cm/s)	14.4	−1	−73	248	0.68
Highest tumor PI	0.90	2	−42	78	0.70
Lowest tumor PI	0.74	3	−49	107	0.59
Tumor color score	26	−4	−71	221	0.89

Inter-CC, interclass correlation coefficient

time-averaged maximum velocity and the color content of tumor scans in extrauterine pelvic tumors. The results of transvaginal color and spectral Doppler examinations of 66 extrauterine pelvic masses made by two observers experienced in ultrasonography (Sladkevicius and myself) were compared. Each observer aimed at obtaining the highest possible Doppler shift from arteries in the wall, septa and solid parts of each tumor. Tumor vascularization was assessed in terms of the 'tumor color score', i.e. the color content of the color Doppler scan as rated for the tumor as a whole by each observer on a visual analog scale. The Doppler measurements were performed at a single examination without any break – i.e. blood flow velocity waveforms were obtained from all sites first by one observer and then by the other, the interval between the two sets of measurements being approximately 25 min, and the total examination time about 50 min. The observers were not present during each other's examinations, and were kept unaware of each other's results until both had made their selection of Doppler shift spectra for analysis. Interobserver agreement (mean difference and limits of agreement, interclass correlation coefficient) was determined for the following variables: peak systolic velocity, time-averaged maximum velocity and pulsatility index in the wall, septum and solid parts of the tumor, the highest peak systolic velocity, the highest time-averaged maximum velocity and the highest and lowest pulsatility index obtained from the tumor as a whole, and color score ratings. The tumors were retrospectively classified according to arbitrarily chosen cut-off limits for the tumor color score, the highest

Table 8 Interobserver agreement in classification of tumors based on cut-off limits for peak systolic velocity (PSV), time-averaged maximum velocity (TAMXV) and tumor color score and on the observer's ability to detect color and to record arterial Doppler shift spectra

	Cohen's Kappa
Highest tumor PSV ≥ 30 cm/s	0.67
Highest tumor TAMXV ≥ 20 cm/s	0.52
Tumor color score ≥ 45	0.66
Color Doppler signals detected	1.0
Arterial Doppler shift spectrum recorded	0.82

tumor time-averaged maximum velocity and the highest tumor peak systolic velocity. Thereafter, interobserver agreement (Cohen's Kappa) was assessed in classifying individual tumors according to the arbitrarily chosen cut-off limits and in detecting color and recording arterial Doppler shift spectra from the tumors. The results are summarized in Tables 7 and 8.

The results in Table 7 show that the two observers seldom recorded the same values for time-averaged maximum velocity or peak systolic velocity, and that they differed considerably in tumor color scores, the ranges between the lower and upper limits of agreement for the percentage differences between the observers being very large. It was to be expected that the reproducibility of Doppler measurements of blood flow velocities in tumor vessels would be unsatisfactory. Most tumors contain many vessels, and it is virtually impossible for two independent observers to sample the same vessels consistently. Moreover, there is the problem of the angle dependence of blood flow velocity measurements. It is also not surprising that the tumor color score ratings differed widely between the two observers, as tumor color score ratings are subjective. Despite the large differences in measurement results between the two observers, some interclass correlation coefficient values were close to 0.75, a value considered to indicate a test to be good enough to allow discrimination between individual subjects or entities (in this case tumors)[24]. However, a satisfactory interclass correlation coefficient (0.89) was obtained only for the tumor color score, indicating that tumor color score alone but none of the other measurement variables allowed good discrimination between the individual tumors in the series.

Interobserver agreement was much better for categorical data than for continuous data, the Kappa values indicating fair to excellent agreement for all the Doppler variables (Table 8). The clinical use of Doppler measurements of the pulsatility index or resistance index in the evaluation of adnexal tumors is based on a classification system whereby tumors with pulsatility index or resistance index values falling below a given cut-off value are classified as likely to be malignant[11,15]. The clinical use of tumor color scores and Doppler measurements of time averaged maximum velocity and peak systolic velocity would also be based on a classification system. Because interobserver agreement in the classification of tumors according to cut-off limits (for the tumor color score and the highest time-averaged maximum velocity and peak systolic velocity) seems to be acceptable, it should be possible to use these Doppler variables as clinical variables with which to characterize extrauterine pelvic masses – at least from the point of view of reproducibility. The sensitivity and specificity of these variables when used as an aid in distinguishing benign from malignant pelvic masses have been described in a recent publication[46]. The color content of the color Doppler tumor scan proved to be the best Doppler variable for distinguishing benignity from malignancy[46].

Our reproducibility study cited above[42] was designed to evaluate the reproducibility of Doppler measurements of blood flow velocities and the color content of color Doppler tumor scans. We had two reasons for studying blood flow velocities and tumor color content instead of blood flow velocity waveform indices: first, in a previous study we had found blood flow velocity to be better than the pulsatility index in differentiating benign and malignant adnexal tumors[12]; second, we suspected the color content of tumor scans to be useful in predicting malignancy (a suspicion that later proved to be true[46]). Thus, it was not the purpose of our reproducibility study[42] to test the reproducibility of pulsatility index measurements; the observers did not try to reproduce each other's pulsatility index values – e.g. by aiming at detecting the highest or lowest pulsatility index of the tumor. Therefore, the large differences in recorded pulsatility index values between the two observers in our study (Table 7) do not necessarily mean that the pulsatility index cannot be reproducibly measured in tumor vessels. For proper evaluation of the interobserver agreement in measurements of pulsatility index in tumors, a different study design would have been necessary. The reason that we did not test intraobserver repeatability of results of Doppler ultrasound examinations of tumors was that we were unable to design a practically feasible study allowing unbiased repeated measurements by the same observer.

Intraobserver repeatability of measurements of pulsatility index, resistance index, peak systolic velocity and time-averaged maximum velocity in benign ovarian tumors was evaluated by Tekay and Jouppila[43]. They found repeatability to be surprisingly good, with intraclass correlation coefficients varying from 0.75 to 0.96 and coefficients of variation from 13 to 33%. However, as only 5 min elapsed between the two measurements made by the same observer, the second measurement might have been biased. Moreover, only two vessels in each tumor were examined.

CONCLUSIONS

Surprisingly little has been published on the reproducibility of gynecological Doppler measurements. Published reports indicate that it is difficult to measure blood flow velocities reproducibly in uterine and ovarian arteries and tumor arteries. The limited reproducibility of Doppler measurements in the uterine and ovarian arteries probably does not allow the detection of small or even moderate physiological differences; only large differences can be expected to be detected. Therefore, the results of studies in which the Doppler technique is used to investigate physiological changes in uterine and ovarian blood circulation must be interpreted with caution.

The clinical use of Doppler variables in the evaluation of adnexal tumors is based on a classification system whereby tumors with values below or above a given cut-off value are classified as likely to be malignant. Interobserver agreement in the classification of extrauterine pelvic tumors according to cut-off limits for time-averaged maximum velocity and peak systolic velocity and the color content of color Doppler tumor scans seems to be good enough to allow the use of these Doppler variables to characterize pelvic masses in a clinical setting. Intraobserver repeatability of measurements of pulsatility index, resistance index, peak systolic velocity and time-averaged maximum velocity in benign adnexal tumors has been evaluated in one study and found to be satisfactory.

References

1. Sladkevicius, P., Valentin, L. and Marsál, K. (1993). Blood flow velocity in the uterine and ovarian arteries during the normal menstrual cycle. *Ultrasound Obstet. Gynecol.*, **3**, 199–208
2. Sladkevicius, P., Valentin, L. and Marsál, K. (1994). Blood flow velocity in the uterine and ovarian arteries during menstruation. *Ultrasound Obstet. Gynecol.*, **4**, 421–7
3. Sladkevicius, P., Valentin, L. and Marsál, K. (1995). Transvaginal gray-scale and Doppler ultrasound examinations of the uterus and ovaries in healthy postmenopausal women. *Ultrasound Obstet. Gynecol.*, **6**, 81–90
4. Valentin, L., Sladkevicius, P., Laurini, R., Söderberg, H. and Marsál, K. (1996). Doppler velocimetry of uteroplacental and luteal circulation in normal first trimester pregnancies. *Am. J. Obstet. Gynecol.*, **174**, 768–75
5. Goswamy, R. K., Williams, G. and Steptoe, P. (1988). Decreased uterine perfusion – a cause of infertility. *Hum. Reprod.*, **3**, 955–9
6. Steer, C. V., Tan, S. L., Mason, B. A. and Campbell, S. (1994). Midluteal phase vaginal color Doppler assessment of uterine artery impedance in a subfertile population. *Fertil. Steril.*, **61**, 53–8
7. Tinkanen, H., Kujansuu, E. and Laippala, P. (1994). Vascular resistance in uterine and ovarian arteries: its association with infertility and the prognosis of fertility. *Eur. J. Obstet. Gynecol. Reprod. Biol.*, **57**, 111–5
8. Kupesic, S. and Kurjak, A. (1993). Uterine and ovarian perfusion during the periovulatory period assessed by transvaginal color Doppler. *Fertil. Steril.*, **60**, 439–43
9. Kurjak, A., Kupesic-Urek, S., Schulman, H. and Zalud, I. (1991). Transvaginal color flow Doppler in the assessment of ovarian and uterine blood flow in infertile women. *Fertil. Steril.*, **56**, 870–3
10. Bourne, T., Campbell, S., Steer, C., Whitehead, M. I. and Collins, W. P. (1989). Transvaginal colour flow imaging: a possible new screening technique for ovarian cancer. *Br. Med. J.*, **299**, 1367–70
11. Kurjak, A., Zalud, I., Jurkovic, D., Alfirevic, Z. and Miljan, M. (1989). Transvaginal color Doppler for the assessment of pelvic circulation. *Acta Obstet. Gynecol. Scand.*, **68**, 131–5
12. Valentin, L., Sladkevicius, P. and Marsál, K. (1994). Limited contribution of Doppler velocimetry to the differential diagnosis of extrauterine pelvic tumors. *Obstet. Gynecol.*, **83**, 425–33
13. Scherjon, S. A., Kok, J. H., Oosting, H. and Zondervan, H. A. (1993). Intra-observer and inter-observer reliability of the PI calculated from pulsed Doppler flow velocity waveforms in three fetal vessels. *Br. J. Obstet. Gynaecol.*, **100**, 134–8
14. Serfontein, G. L. and Jaroszewics, A. M. (1978). Estimation of gestational age at birth: comparison of two methods. *Arch. Dis. Child.*, **53**, 509–11
15. Bland, J. M. and Altman, D. G. (1986). Statistical methods for assessing agreement between two methods of clinical measurement. *Lancet*, **1**, 307–10
16. Bourne, T. H., Campbell, S., Steer, C. V., Royston, P., Whitehead, M. I. and Collins, W. P.

(1991). Detection of endometrial cancer by transvaginal ultrasonography with color flow imaging and blood flow analysis: a preliminary report. *Gynecol. Oncol.*, **40**, 253–9

17. Steer, C. V., Campbell, S., Pampiglione, J. S., Kingsland, C. R., Mason, B. A. and Collins, W. P. (1990). Transvaginal colour flow imaging of the uterine arteries during the ovarian and menstrual cycles. *Hum. Reprod.*, **5**, 391–5

18. Mercé, L. T., Garcés, D., Barco, M. J., and de la Fuente, F. (1992). Intraovarian Doppler velocimetry in ovulatory, dysovulatory and anovulatory cycles. *Ultrasound Obstet. Gynecol.*, **2**, 197–202

19. Collins, W., Jurkovic, D., Bourne, T., Kurjak, A. and Campbell, S. (1991). Ovarian morphology, endocrine function and intra-follicular blood flow during the peri-ovulatory period. *Hum. Reprod.*, **3**, 319–24

20. Bourne, T. H., Jurkovic, D., Waterstone, J., Campbell, S. and Collins, W. P. (1991). Intra-follicular blood flow during human ovulation. *Ultrasound Obstet. Gynecol.*, **1**, 53–9

21. Long, M. G., Boultbee, J. E., Hanson, M. E. and Begent, R. H. J. (1989). Doppler time velocity waveform studies of the uterine artery and uterus. *Br. J. Obstet. Gynaecol.*, **86**, 588–93

22. Bland, J. M. and Altman, D. G. (1990). A note on the use of the intraclass correlation coefficient in the evaluation of agreement between two methods of measurement. *Comput. Biol. Med.*, **20**, 337–40

23. Brennan, P. and Silman, A. (1992). Statistical methods for assessing observer variability in clinical measures. *Br. Med. J.*, **304**, 1491–4

24. Burdock, E. I., Fleiss, J. L. and Hardesty, A. S. (1963). A new view of interobserver agreement. *Pers. Psychol.*, **16**, 373–84

25. Kramer, M. S. and Feinstein, A. R. (1981). Clinical biostatistics. The biostatistics of concordance. *Clin. Pharmacol. Ther.*, **29**, 111–23

26. Cohen, J. (1960). A coefficient of agreement for nominal scales. *Educ. Psychol. Measur.*, **20**, 37–46

27. Gudmundsson, S. and Marsál, K. (1988). Umbilical artery and uteroplacental blood flow velocity waveforms in normal pregnancy – a cross sectional study. *Acta Obstet. Gynecol. Scand.*, **67**, 347–54

28. Lingman, G. and Marsál, K. (1986). Fetal central blood circulation in the third trimester of normal pregnancy. Longitudinal study. II. Aortic blood flow velocity waveform. *Early Hum. Dev.*, **13**, 151–9

29. Thompson, R. S., Trudinger, B. J. and Cook, C. M. (1986). A comparison of Doppler ultrasound waveform indices in the umbilical artery. I. Indices derived from the maximum velocity waveform. *Ultrasound Med. Biol.*, **12**, 835–44

30. Mires, G., Dempster, J., Patel, N. B. and Crawford, J. W. (1987). The effect of fetal heart rate on umbilical artery blood flow velocity waveforms. *Br. J. Obstet. Gynaecol.*, **96**, 665–9

31. Mulders, L. G. M., Muijers, G. J. J. M., Jongsma, H. W., Nijhuis, J. G. and Hein, P. R. (1986). The umbilical artery blood flow velocity waveform in relation to fetal breathing movements, fetal heart rate and fetal behavioural states in normal pregnancy at 37–39 weeks. *Early Hum. Dev.*, **14**, 283–93

32. Cibils, L. A. (1967). Contractility of the non-pregnant human uterus. *Obstet. Gynecol.*, **30**, 441–61

33. Hein, P. R., Eskes, T. K. A. B., Stolte, L. A. M., Braaksma, J. T., Janssens, J. and v.d. Hoek, J. B. (1973). The influence of steroids on uterine motility in the nonpregnant human uterus. In Josimovich, J. B. (ed.) *Uterine Contraction: Side Effects of Steroidal Contraceptives*, pp. 107–28. (New York: A. Wiley Interscience Series)

34. Farquar, C. M., Rae, T., Thomas, D. C., Wadsworth, J. and Beard, R. W. (1989). Doppler ultrasound in the nonpregnant pelvis. *J. Ultrasound Med.*, **8**, 451–7

35. Sladkevicius, P. and Valentin, L. (1995). Reproducibility of Doppler measurements of blood flow velocities in the uterine and ovarian arteries in premenopausal women. *J. Ultrasound Med. Biol.*, **21**, 313–9

36. Sladkevicius, P. and Valentin, L. (1995). Reproducibility of Doppler measurements of blood flow velocities in the uterine and ovarian arteries in postmenopausal women. *Eur. J. Ultrasound*, **2**, 3–9

37. Tekay, A. and Jouppila, P. (1996). Intraobserver reproducibility of transvaginal Doppler measurements in uterine and intraovarian arteries in regularly menstruating women. *Ultrasound Obstet. Gynecol.*, **7**, 129–34

38. Steer, C. V., Williams, J., Zaidi, J., Campbell, S. and Tan, S. L. (1995). Intra-observer, interobserver, interultrasound transducer and inter-cycle variation in colour Doppler assessment of uterine artery impedance. *Hum. Reprod.*, **10**, 479–81

39. Tinkanen, H. and Kujansuu, E. (1995). The reproducibility of the Doppler ultrasound measurement of uterine artery vascular resistance. *Gynecol. Obstet. Invest.*, **39**, 188–91

40. Sladkevicius, P. (1994). *Doppler ultrasound studies in gynaecology*. Thesis, Lund University, Lund, Sweden

41. Bourne, T. H. (1991). Transvaginal Doppler in gynecology. *Ultrasound Obstet. Gynecol.*, **1**, 359–73

42. Sladkevicius, P. and Valentin, L. (1995). Inter-observer agreement in the results of Doppler

examinations of extrauterine pelvic tumors. *Ultrasound Obstet. Gynecol.*, **6**, 91–6

43. Tekay, A. and Jouppila, P. (1997). Intraobserver variation in transvaginal Doppler blood flow measurements in benign ovarian tumors. *Ultrasound Obstet. Gynecol.*, **9**, 120–4

44. Weiner, Z., Thaler, I., Beck, D., Rottem, S., Deutsch, M. and Brandes, J. M. (1992). Differentiating malignant from benign ovarian tumors with transvaginal color flow imaging. *Obstet. Gynecol.*, **79**, 159–62

45. Kurjak, A. and Predanic, M. (1992). New scoring system for prediction of ovarian malignancy based on transvaginal color Doppler sonography. *J. Ultrasound Med.*, **11**, 631–8

46. Valentin, L. (1997). Gray scale sonography, subjective evaluation of the color Doppler image and measurement of blood flow velocity for distinguishing benign and malignant tumors of suspected adnexal origin. *Eur. J. Obstet. Gynecol. Reprod. Biol.*, **72**, 63–72

Index